To Bob
You can feel elated that your life has truly
been worthwhile, you have given the world the blessing
to be able to be here for a good time *and* a long time.

To Siimon
A true visionary, friend and a man of unquestionable
principle.

Disclaimer

Please note that medicine is referred to in this book as the 'practise of medicine' because it requires constant reeducation and re-evaluation to maintain proficiency and accuracy. The data presented in this book include research on anti-ageing therapeutics written by the best and brightest minds and published by some of the most authoritative texts and journals in the world. But in less than five years from now, we will know twice as much about anti-ageing medicine and biomedical technology as we do today, and 10 years from now we will have more than five times as much knowledge of this subject.

Because of the ever-expanding knowledge of medicine, the most any author can hope to do is to wisely and prudently put forth theory and practice as best as it is currently known. In preparation of this text, the editorial staff reviewed scores of published reports, hundreds of books, and interviewed many of the world's leading anti-ageing researchers and scientists. However, do not assume the material in this book to be 100 per cent correct or safe. It is *not*! This book is not intended to provide medical advice, nor is it to be used as a substitute for advice from your own physician. At best, this book is meant to be an educational resource to guide your personal quest toward enhanced health and longevity. If you wish to initiate any of the programs or therapies described in this book, you *must* consult and work in partnership with a knowledgeable physician before doing so.

Perhaps some day, as Woody Allen wrote in the movie *Sleeper*, we will find that the true keys to health and longevity are hot fudge sundaes and smoking cigars. But for now, we can only rely on the vast preponderance of research, scientific opinion and clinical experience of the individuals whose groundbreaking work helped to fill the pages of this book.

The Anti-ageing Diet:

How to look and feel 20 years younger no matter what your age

by
Brian Sher
Dr Robert Goldman & Dr Ronald Klatz
with
John Gearon

Published by
REDWOOD PUBLISHING
Suite 805, 3 Waverley St, Bondi Junction 2022
Sydney

briansher@bigpond.com.au

First published 2000
Copyright © Brian Sher 2000

National Library of Australia
Cataloguing-in-publication data:

    Sher, Brian
    The Anti-Ageing Diet

    ISBN

    1. Health. 2. Longevity 3. Wellbeing.

Cover by Cherry Design
Typeset by Midland Typesetters
Printed by McPherson's Printing Group

About the authors

Brian Sher

Educated in business and marketing from the University of New South Wales, Brian is one of Australia's most successful marketing consultants, publishers, entrepreneurs, authors and speakers. Director and founder of Australia's first preventative medicine and anti-ageing clinic, he has consulted to more than 1000 business, and is a sought-after business coach charging more than $2000 per hour for his time. His recent book *What Rich People Know and Desperately Want to Keep a Secret* is an Australia best seller soon to be launched in the United States market.

Dr Robert Goldman

Along with being a scientist, surgeon, inventor, researcher, entrepreneur and author, he is a former world champion strength athlete, holding more than 20 world records. He is recognised as a world expert on drug testing and anabolic steroids, and has helped establish international standards in those areas. He has been awarded many patents for his inventions and is the co-founder with Dr Ronald Klatz of the American Academy of Anti-Ageing Medicine, and is Chairman of the Board and the founder and President of the National Academy of Sports Medicine.

Dr Ronald Klatz

One of the world's foremost authorities on preventative/ longevity medicine, he is Senior Medical Editor at Longevity Magazine, founder and President of the American Longevity

Research Institute, co-founder of the National Academy of Sports Medicine and founder of the American Academy of Anti-Ageing Medicine, and author of many previous books and articles. He is board-certified by the American Osteopathic Board of Family Practice, the American Osteopathy Academy of Sports Medicine and the Academy of Sports Physicians.

John Gearon

John has extensive expertise in the fields of Exercise Physiology and Human Nutrition for the past 15 years. He is involved in the fields of Psychological Transformations as a Master Neuro-Linguistic Practitioner, Time Line Therapist and Peak Performance Results Coach, and Lifestyle Director for Redwood, Australia's leading Anti-Ageing Clinic responsible for the physical, nutritional and psychological protocols.

A lecturer throughout Australia, he conducts seminars and keynote speeches and is the author of numerous magazine articles. He is a consultant to the Australian Military Defence Force for its physical training equipment and elite conditioning programs, and a former professional ironman triathlete who has competed in more than 250 triathlons and ironman-length races, including the Hawaiian Ironman Triathlon World Championships.

Contents

Why You Should Hate the Word Diet!

Introduction

100% GUARANTEE: NOT JUST ANOTHER DIET BOOK!

Thank you for purchasing this book. Reading and understanding its contents will without doubt change your life forever.

The information it contains is so amazing and so powerful, that by following **The Anti-ageing Diet** you will gain an additional 10, 20 or maybe 30 years of youthful functional living, free of disease and ill health. This is truly a worthwhile endeavour for any person to strive for.

PERMANENTLY AND NATURALLY REVERSE AGEING – FROM THE INSIDE OUT

The Anti-ageing Diet is not just another diet book.

If you have bought this book expecting just another twist on weight loss or bowel cleansing to keep you healthy, you will be disappointed.

If, however, you are seeking real, true knowledge to help you break through all the clutter and confusion, you will find this book exciting, stimulating and most of all empowering, allowing you to take control of your health once and for all.

Finally, you will gain a true understanding of how to look and feel young all through your life, along the way learning about the many wonderful natural substances and medical breakthroughs that will help you live a long, healthy vibrant life.

I have no doubt you will be ecstatic, as I was, to discover this new natural medical science now available to all of us today.

A FOOL-PROOF DIET

The Anti-ageing Diet is also not a diet you can fail on.

If you do indeed make a decision and a commitment to follow this diet, the great news is you can eat just about anything you like, but not all the time.

If you feel like chocolate, feel free — have it. If you feel like a glass of wine or beer — have it. If you feel like ice cream or coffee — have it . . . but you can now put it all in perspective.

The great news about the **Anti-ageing Diet** is that you can still indulge yourself in things you like that are 'bad' for you, as long as this is only 5% of the time. In other words, you cannot blow your **Anti-ageing Diet** as long as 95% of the time you do it right.

This attitude of balance between no deprivation and preserving your long-term health is very important in being able to succeed on your **Anti-ageing Diet** throughout your life. Indulging yourself 5% of the time allows you to feel good about yourself and allows you never to feel like you are missing out in life, as long as bad eating, drinking or other bad habits don't become exactly that — bad habits.

THE ULTIMATE DIET – THAT WILL SAVE YOUR LIFE

Having said that, I am secure in claiming this is the ultimate diet book, as if offers real, manageable and totally flexible options to everyone and anyone.

Please note: We have used the word **Diet** here in a much different context to most other books that suggest a certain regime of eating to reduce, or control, body weight.

The Anti-ageing Diet is much, much more important than that. It has far more important consequences for your long-term health than shedding a few extra kilos.

The Anti-ageing Diet is the last diet you will ever need to go on.

It is a sensible guide to not only how you eat, but how you can take advantage of the new natural medical alternatives that are now available. These will not only provide you with optimal and lasting health but could save your life, or even better save you from many years of unnecessary disease, pain and suffering in your later years. Nobody – and I mean nobody – wants to find themselves permanently in an aged-care home, with the loss of their independence and dignity. But this is the way many, many people end their lives, sadly. DO NOT LET THIS HAPPEN TO YOU.

Until now the word Anti-ageing has been associated with cosmetic improvements or external substances applied to the skin to 'hide' the signs of ageing, as it has been the belief up until now that ageing cannot be reversed or slowed, except cosmetically.

This is all set to change.

NATURAL BEAUTY FROM THE INSIDE OUT

For the first time in history, science is providing us with breakthroughs. There are now proven methods and natural substances that are available to slow, stop and even reverse the ageing process, *from the inside out*.

With medical knowledge in this area doubling every 3–5 years, this is just the beginning.

The science of Anti-ageing together with genetic engineering will see some remarkable breakthroughs in the fight against ageing and disease. These new discoveries will dwarf many of the greatest discoveries and inventions made by mankind to this day.

We are indeed entering a brand-new era of medicine and science so advanced and so exciting that it promises to deliver immortality and eternal youth, previously just the dream of 'mad' or deranged scientists.

KNOWLEDGE IS POWER!

And with this new knowledge we now have, we will be in a far better position to dispel much of the confusion about the correct choices to make. We will be in a superior position to make the right choices for ourselves and the quality of our own lives, keeping those decisions within our own grasp, not relinquishing them to the medical fraternity.

As you turn the page, you are about to start an exciting and far-ranging journey like no other you've ever encountered before. This journey and the new decisions you will make about what you eat, drink and how to live your daily life will have an impact on you and those around you, forever.

With this new knowledge comes a greater responsibility – to help others less fortunate than ourselves, encouraging them to educate themselves in this knowledge and giving them back control over their own lives and health.

This book could have been titled . . .

FORGET ABOUT MONEY . . . WITHOUT HEALTH YOU ARE BANKRUPT ANYWAY.

This is the real message of the book . . . have a great deal of knowledge about your health and what you put into your body. Your health is the most important asset you have. Unlike any other asset, however, if your health is lost it is irreplaceable, no matter how much money you have.

HOSPITALS AND NURSING HOMES ARE FULL OF SELF-INFLICTED DISEASES

Who says that growing older has to mean the increased incidence of sickness? Many diseases, including heart disease, cancer, arthritis, osteoporosis, Alzheimer's and many more, are self-inflicted and could be termed Westerners' Disease.

There is a direct link between the way we live in western society and the early onset of many of these diseases. Our hospitals and nursing homes are full to capacity with people who, given the right knowledge 20, 10 or even 5 years ago, could have delayed or avoided having to spend the rest of their lives in a dysfunctional state.

The onset of poor health has far more serious implications and impact than just the contracting of diseases alone. Older people who have lost their health, mobility independence by being confined to a hospital bed or nursing home lose the most important of all human emotions . . . pride and dignity.

This is the real tragedy, as it leads quickly to serious depression and total loss of willingness to live. This need not be the case.

If we begin to realise as early as possible – today, for example – that if we want to avoid this happening to us, we cannot rely on doctors to save us when we get sick, or by some chance or good genetic make up.

We need to start living a new, sensible lifestyle, which starts with the practising of this **Anti-ageing Diet**.

Do not think it won't happen to you ... old people were once young, too.

They never imagined living the last years of their life like that, either. But when the day does come, wishing they could change it won't help.

YOUR VERY OWN RUBBISH DUMP

I am often amazed by people who maintain their house or car better than they maintain their bodies. If you compare the way many people treat their bodies to the way they treat their houses, they would be living in a dirty, disease-ridden rubbish dump with all the toxins, pollutants and other biologically mismatched 'food' they dump into their bodies.

And it shows. If you are sick, overweight or looking old, just stop and look at your lifestyle and I am sure there's an explanation in that somewhere.

Some people are just born genetically lucky (or unlucky) – that's life – but 90% of the time ageing badly and suffering disease has got direct links to your environment and how you are currently living your life.

So congratulate yourself. You are amongst the first people

in Australia, or indeed the world, to discover the new era of Anti-ageing medicine that will help you stay young, fit and healthy well into your 70s, 80s and 90s and beyond.

A SIMPLE EXPLANATION OF HOW TO STAY YOUNG

I have read many books on health and medicine, and found many of them to be too technical or detailed to digest the information into something useable and practical.

This book is purposely different. It was written for the non-medical everyday person to try to make sense of all the marketing hype. It will help you remove the confusion, as the information has been simplified into easy-to-read principles that can be understood and applied in our daily lives.

Your health is a serious issue. The body in all its millions of functions is highly complex, so much so that nobody has a complete understanding of how it all works. In many cases, even the most highly trained doctors can only speculate or guess exactly how the body functions.

The Anti-ageing Diet is not meant to be the definitive guide to all health issues, but a practical, easy-to-read guide to help you understand the many complex issues with regard to your accelerated ageing, and the important choices you make on a daily basis.

BEAUTY IS SKIN DEEP

You do not have to be a doctor to diagnose if someone is sick or healthy. Just look at their skin.

The skin, especially on the face and around the eyes, will tell you instantly about the state of a person's biological health. The colour, texture, bags around the eyes, the elasticity, fat deposits on cheeks and chin, wrinkles, spots, blemishes and so on tell a very revealing story about the state of their health. Now, have another look in the mirror and what do you see?

Billions of dollars are spent each year by women around the world on make-up, skin creams and cosmetic interventions in an attempt to keep their skin looking younger and ward off the signs of ageing – dry, wrinkled, inelastic skin covered with 'age spots' and pallor.

The outstanding news for these women (and also men) is that the skin is simply another organ of the body. The health and age of your skin is a great indicator as to the health and biological age of your other organs and your entire body.

The Anti-ageing Diet will not only help you feel younger on the inside, giving you more life, health and energy, but as your skin is your body's largest organ it will also have dramatic effects on how young you look, too.

No matter what your chronological age or genetic make up, following **The Anti-ageing Diet** will without doubt help keep you not only feeling 20 years younger but looking 20 years younger, too.

Some people may still disagree, and say that's impossible. Yet it has been scientifically proven that the recommendations outlined in this book have dramatic effects on the rate at which you age.

By keeping your body's internal biochemistry stable and healthy, allowing your body to commit its energy and resources into cell repair and rejuvenation from the inside (increasing the number of new cells that are being produced relative to those that are dying), you will stay young and healthy.

If this high rate of rejuvenation continues at a cellular level for longer periods of time, the entire body, including the skin, will remain young in appearance and function.

A BEAUTIFUL YOUNG SKIN WILL ALSO SAVE YOUR LIFE

This is a truly remarkable breakthrough for women and skin care, and promises to revolutionise the entire way women think about their skin.

The fact alone that a healthy internal body will mean a healthy younger skin will also indirectly help save many lives.

When Anti-ageing (from the inside) gains mass appeal over the next few years, and women all over the world realise beauty and preventative health are one and the same thing, they will begin to follow these daily practices for no other reason but to keep their skin young.

These same practices will be the very things that will save their lives, by preventing life-threatening diseases from rapid ageing.

Their only motivation may be to have younger-looking skin, but the result will be improved general health, which is not a bad result.

Section 1

STOPPING THE CLOCK

'The problem with Youth is it's wasted on the young!'

Forget ageing gracefully.

If we were really honest with ourselves, very few of us would choose to grow old.

For some, this choice would be pure vanity, but for most it is the fear of what age brings that frightens us about old age – loss of function, independence and usefulness.

Let's face it – who wouldn't want to be as fit and vital at 75 as they were at 35?

If you could have one wish, what would it be? When asked, most people would say 'Eternal youth, of course'. But what people wish for and what they get are two separate issues.

Still, today, with all our wisdom and technology, people are growing older. Noticeable ageing starts sometime in our mid twenties and begins to bring on minor ailments from weight gain, loss of memory, loss of energy and vitality, loss of hair and skin elasticity, to major disability, deformity, pain, disease and sorrow on a wholesale basis.

Youth and good looks have a high priority in our society (just open any glossy magazine if you need to be convinced of this) and old people are regarded as a liability, something to be pitied, and less than useful.

This, however, need not be the case.

Growing older does not have to automatically bring with it decrepitude and uselessness, and all the connotations associated with this in western society. Age should be cherished as one might appreciate a vintage automobile or antique painting, but, sadly, as people our value to society decreases as we age.

Indeed, for this reason, for thousands of years the fear of growing old has caused man to dream of the prevention of ageing, and it has always been the Holy Grail of medicine and science.

But now, thanks to some remarkable breakthroughs in science and their practical application in what we have coined in this new book '**The Anti-ageing Diet**' (the science of keeping young and healthy from the inside out), what was once just a dream is now an awesome reality.

Anti-ageing not only exists, it is clinically and medically proven to work, and will soon be as popular as the Internet revolution.

Some of the world's finest medical research institutions (like Harvard, Stanford and UCLA medical school) have undertaken extensive studies revealing foods, nutrients, exercise, natural drugs and body maintenance systems administered in exactly the right amounts can keep people younger as we know it today for decades longer than previously thought.

YOU WILL ONLY BE MIDDLE-AGED WHEN YOU ARE 80

In fact, the current evidence suggests that it should be absolutely possible for humans to stay middle-aged until 70 or 80 years of age, and then go on to live healthy vibrant lives to their 120th birthday and beyond.

Most people reading this now can fully expect 100+ lifespans. In fact, within the next 30 years we can expect to see lifespans of 120–130 years in people with their physical states sound and intact with sharp and acute mental capacities.

WE CAN STOP THE CLOCK!

The time has come and it is now here.

We can stop the clock, or at least slow it down in most cases. New metabolic and nutritional approaches, together with proper mass education and lifestyle changes, can help us reverse the wholesale DNA and tissue damage taking place through lack of awareness and self-abuse. Many of the causes and terrible effects of rapid ageing and body deterioration are self-induced and can be reversed or avoided with **The Anti-ageing Diet**.

Doctor Ronald Klatz, the President of the American Academy of the Anti-ageing Medicine says, 'Forget growing old gracefully. We're interested in not growing old. Anti-ageing specialists hold the position that "**ageing is not inevitable**".'

Dr Klatz is, of course, not referring to **chronological age** or the number of birthdays you accumulate. What he and other Anti-ageing specialists are referring to is your **biological age**. In other words, what is important is not your age but the relative health of your body and its ability to function normally and fight of the effects of disease.

'We plan on helping our patients stay young for as long as science and technology will allow. Many of the disorders we used to think were part and parcel of old age can be corrected.'

THERE'S NOTHING WRONG WITH AGEING EXCEPT . . .

To understand the concept of Anti-ageing, realise that, with the exception of infection and some childhood disorders, the vast majority of degenerative diseases share but one common characteristic − ageing itself.

With ageing, apart from the loss of our youthful appearance, the main concern for most people is that our functions − activities, memory and creativity we once enjoyed − begin to deteriorate. We experience a sharp decline in our immune defence system, leaving us more susceptible to disease, sapping us of energy, vitality and earning capacity on which we depend to survive.

Until now we have accepted diseases of ageing as our fate, justified as a normal part of life. We have been led to believe that a lower quality of life is inevitable once we start to approach our 50s and 60s.

Diseases such as cancer, heart disease, stroke, osteoporosis, loss of memory and sexual desire, diabetes, Alzheimer's, fatigue, arthritis, Parkinson's disease, obesity and other diseases are on the increase despite the millions of dollars that are being spent each year by drug and research companies to find cures.

Scientists more recently, however, have discovered a

single, yet common, thread to all of these diseases – ageing! The older we are the greater the likelihood of our health being affected by disease

This is now set to change, with a boom in a new and exciting medical specialty – Anti-ageing medicine and the everyday practice of this revolutionary **The Anti-ageing Diet**.

WHAT IS THE ANTI-AGEING DIET?

With this new, powerful knowledge on how the human body ages, we can begin to practise and live a longer healthier life by focusing on reversing the internal ageing process itself. And on preventing, rejuvenating and boosting the most powerful anti-disease system know to man – our own immune system. The great bonus we get from this discipline is that we not only *feel* healthier and younger for the rest of our lives, we *look* younger, too.

Anti-ageing medicine using every day practise of **The Anti-ageing Diet** has scientifically proven that, by using safe, natural foods, natural nutrients, exercise, stress relief and superhormones, age and disease can be slowed and even reversed by as much as 20 years.

Our brains, organs and muscles can quickly be regenerated and strengthened back to youthful levels, which in turn boosts our energy, vitality and sharpness of mind.

This is indeed one of the most remarkable breakthroughs this decade, to help fight disease, extend the quality of human life and keep people looking and feeling young, healthy and vibrant.

For people who are already following **The Anti-ageing Diet** it is proving to be amazingly effective, yet this new knowledge has so much more to offer. If one considers that medical knowledge in this area is doubling every 3–5 years, then it is obvious its impact on society in the next decade will be nothing short of incredible.

THE STAYING-YOUNG EXPLOSION

Baby boomers today are starting to hit their 50s, yet are not prepared to grow old. Unlike previous generations, age is not something that they are prepared to accept nor are they willing to grow old gracefully.

In Australia, one in five of us already visits alternative health therapists and are spending around $400 million pa. for the privilege. (*Natural Health p42 May 1998). This figure is the estimate for alternative health services only, and does not include income spent on health products and natural alternatives. Combining this together, the figure may be as high as $1 billion. Worldwide, this market may be estimated at around $40 billion already.

Over the next 20 years, as the Baby Boomers hit their 50s, 60s,and 70s, this figure is expected to explode.

TRADITIONAL MEDICINE – A LOSING BATTLE

The traditional health system is in crisis.

We are fighting a losing battle by focusing on the symptoms and not the cause of disease. People believe that it is OK to eat drink and abuse our bodies, and that there will be a doctor available free of charge in every suburb with a 'fix-it' pill when we eventually (and we will) get sick.

With the growing realisation of its inherent shortcomings

(treating the symptoms and not the cause), traditional medicine it is facing the inevitable – the inability to cope with the ever-increasing volume and costs of treatment, yet still is not providing answers.

This being the reality, more and more people will have no option, if they wish to remain healthy, and will be forced to take responsibility in full or in part for their own health, not by taking out health insurance but by seeking prevention rather than cure.

YOU OR THE PERSON NEXT TO YOU WILL GET CANCER!

With literally billions of dollars being spent on medical research and treatments, it is no surprise to discover the medical establishment is failing. Consider the following facts:

As it stands now, 1/3 of Australians will get some form of cancer at some point in their lives, and by the year 2000 this figure is expected to increase to 1/2.

Nearly 60% of people over 65 experience high blood pressure and 33% have heart disease. 45% of the elderly are on prescription drugs, suffering ailments ranging from arthritis to hypertension to glaucoma. (*Natural Health p42 May 1998).

Considering the above, unless immediate changes are made, most people approaching the ages of 40, 50, and 60 can expect to experience some form of disease, such as cancer, arthritis, osteoporosis, arteriosclerosis, heart disease, Alzheimer's, loss of sexual drive, loss of mobility, strength and agility, loss of memory and vitality, diabetes, stroke, pneumonia, Parkinson's disease, etc.

THE NATION'S HEALTH – A POLITICIAN'S NIGHTMARE

With the ageing of the Baby Boomers – the largest portion of our population – and the ever-increasing demand and cost of medical treatments for those that are ageing with sickness, health care as a political issue will become increasingly important and already is at a flash point.

Due to this demographic reaching this critical age and our reliance on government-sponsored health care, governments, no matter whether they be right or left wing, will be unable to stop the cost blowout and be unable to fund these ever-rising costs. They, too, will soon be desperately looking for alternatives and will sooner or later need to come to the realisation of redirecting resources into preventing disease rather than trying to cure it.

BIG STAKES!

Consider the US example of saving $3 billion a year by reducing the average nursing home stay by just one month. A further saving of $40 billion per year could be achieved should the onset of Alzheimer's be delayed by an average of 5 years.

You will see the inevitable attraction of governments to this medicine, when they discover the huge cost savings it can create. Traditional medicine has helped keep people alive some 30 years longer this century, but this has not come without a cost. It has been equally unsuccessful in offering them something much more important – a better quality of life.

Unfortunately, even though people are living longer, they

are spending many of their middle to later years fighting the effect of disease and are in poor health.

THE GOOD NEWS – AGEING IS NOT INEVITABLE

All this is set to change, as people realise that age-related disease is not inevitable and that science now offers a real, exciting and tangible alternative.

The future will need to see people changing their attitude toward medicine and making visits to their Anti-ageing adviser to ensure they remain healthy, rather than visit their doctors only when they become sick.

Contrary to popular belief, these diseases are not inevitable and can be avoided or reversed with current Anti-ageing medicine. Anti-ageing technology today is so advanced it has the ability to reverse the effects of ageing and keep an individual's biological age some 20 years younger than their chronological age, and in so doing keep diseases of affluence in check.

One point to highlight is that the ultimate promise of Anti-ageing is not necessarily to help people to live longer – traditional medicine has succeeded at that – but to offer people something that money cannot buy: **both health and longevity**.

OUR BODIES ARE OBSOLETE MODELS

According to Dr Vincent Giampapa at the Longevity Institute in NJ, as a species we were genetically complete approximately 1 million years ago. In other words, our bodies have been designed, if you like, to deal with life as it was at that time.

Logic will tell you that times were very different back then. There was no industrialisation, mechanisation or technology. To eat, live and survive, we would gather grain and fruits between hunting on foot, occasionally catching small animals to eat. Our diets were primarily vegetarian, and we gained plenty of exercise (walking and running) while hunting and having the occasional meal of animal protein. The most stress man may have encountered back then was the threat of being chased or killed by a dinosaur.

Today, to live and survive, most of us need do very little physical work in our office jobs to earn a living. We do not need to worry about food until we are hungry, with a vast array of food readily available on every street corner, most with very little nutritional value.

In order to achieve optimal health, we need to consider the way we live in light of the above. In the short term, our bodies can take much abuse and be forgiving, but after many years of stress, environmental pollution and poor-quality foods, it will accelerate our ageing and the onset of disease.

We must see our bodies as a finely tuned, high-performance race car speeding around a wet track. It does not take much for it to veer off course, and there are dangerous obstacles all around – in the form of degenerative diseases.

When we are young we are approximately 80% muscle and lean tissue and 20% fat. With each decade that passes (if we do not maintain our bodies as suggested) we have more of our lean muscle replaced by fat, so that by the time we are in our 70s our ratio is more like 50/50.

IS YOUR SALAD REALLY HEALTHY?

Dr Ronald Klatz, in his book 7 Anti-ageing Secrets, explains the following: Our bodies have not changed much, especially in the last century, but the genetic quality of the food we eat has been altered radically.

The red tomato in your salad today we mistakenly believe is healthy and nutritious. It unfortunately is the product of numerous chemical reactions, preservatives, dyes, freezing and other storage methods. A lean cut of red meat or chicken contains a variety of antibiotics, growth hormones and steroids.

All you have to do is take a trip to a rural part of southern Europe and you will quickly note how extraordinarily different truly fresh fish, fruit and vegetables taste. The high quality of fresh, natural foods account in large part for why populations in southern Spain and Italy have the longest life spans for all of Europe despite the population's consumption of large amounts of oils, meat and dairy products.

The modern world is inundated with totally processed, manufactured and nutritionally deficient foods, creating a highly imbalanced daily nutritional intake. They contain so many environmental toxins, many so new we have yet to discover their ultimate effects on human health.

WHO IS RICHER?

We must ask ourselves why, when we live in countries with some of the highest levels of technology and education with millions spent daily in our health systems, our cumulative health is so poor. Yet there are cultures in the world that are uneducated and live in far less hygienic and comfortable environments but which enjoy longer, more productive lives.

Amongst these cultures are the Vilcabambas who live in the Andes mountains in Ecuador; the Bilcabamba of Peru; the Abkahasians on the eastern shores of the Black Sea; and the Hunzas in the Himalayas in Northern Peru. The elderly in these societies live long and productive lives. They are respected and honoured and old age does not have the connotations of decrepitude and uselessness that it does in western society.

One of the biggest factors that affect the life span of the elderly in these villages is their diet.

The conclusion is that people who live the longest in the world eat simple diets, eating the same food consistently throughout their lives. Their meals are low in calories, fats and animal protein. In addition, people of these communities lead relatively uneventful, stress-free lives.

LET THE MAYOR WORRY!

It has been reported that the Hunzas lead a completely stress-free life and enjoy much social support from their families and community. The Hunza population is divided into villages; each village is led by its own mayor. Any time there is a problem, people bring it to the attention of the mayor, and he takes care of it so no one else has to worry. While the citizens of his village live to 95 or 100 years before they begin to think of themselves as elders, the mayors of the village rarely live past the age of 60!

Also, we must account for the fact that these long-living cultures include much physical exercise in their lives. Because they live in the mountains and continue to work until a late stage in their lives their metabolism, circulation and digestive systems are in good order. Because of their low cholesterol and blood pressure, heart disease and cancer are practically unheard of.

On the other hand, we also have a lot to learn from societies with the shortest life expectancies. These include Eskimos, Laplanders, Greenlanders and Russian Kurds. They have an average life expectancy of approximately 30 years. All are primarily meat eaters and live in cold climates where vegetables are hard to find.

WHY DO WE AGE?

To best explain the Anti-ageing methodologies and the solid reasoning behind the creation of the now world famous **Anti-Ageing Diet**, let us first outline the known 4 major theories of ageing.

• **THE WEAR AND TEAR THEORY**
This theory simply states the body and its cells are damaged by over-use and abuse. The wearing out of vital organs, gland and cellular structures is largely the result of stress. Stress speeds up our ageing clock.

Stress includes the daily anxieties from the fast-paced life we live and the demands placed on our time and focus. Stress also results from a poor diet and environmental toxins – high in processed foods, chemicals, sugars, acids, fats and artificial substances. These wreak havoc on our biochemistry and hormones by breaking down important proteins and gene-repairing mechanisms and reduce circulation in areas such as the digestive system.

• FREE-RADICAL THEORY

Normal cell activity produces waste products. Along with environmental pollutants, poor nutrition and digestion are highly toxic to cells and DNA. These unwanted biochemicals, called free radicals, are generated by the breakdown of oxygen (oxidisation) and cause damage to the energy sites in the cells – the mitochondria. This process is similar to metals that rust, slowly weaken and get eaten away.

• NEUROENDOCRINE THEORY

This is the decline of the nervous and endocrine systems and lessening of their ability to regulate and integrate the body's key activities. Key hormones such as melatonin, HGH, IGF-1 and DHEA decline by around 10% per decade. Decreased hormonal levels result in a body-wide imbalance that decreases the immune system, strength, metabolism and sexual functions.

• GENETIC CONTROL THEORY

This theory states that the body's own genes are genetically programmed to stop repair and maintenance after a pre-determined time. Scientists have discovered that specific genes are related to specific age-related illnesses. These genetic weaknesses predispose individuals to develop certain disorders by making them more vulnerable to outside influences such as stress, poor nutrition, and environmental toxins.

In total there are approximately 18 theories of ageing, however these four are the most widely known and accepted theories.

SO WHICH IS THE MOST ACCURATE EXPLANATION OF AGEING?

The facts seem to show that no one theory on its own can fully explain why we age. Scientists and Anti-ageing specialists seem to agree that ageing is caused in part by all of these factors, and to successfully stave off the effects of ageing, Anti-ageing medicine has developed a complete program – **The Anti-ageing Diet** – which address all of these factors individually.

HOW DOES THE BODY WORK SO EFFICIENTLY?

In order to understand ageing we first need to quickly review our biology lessons to recall why and how the body functions. Our complete bodily functions (and there are thousands of these each minute), depend on a series of highly complex and critically timed chemical reactions in order to function 'normally'. Every cell in your body depends on hundreds of chemical messages and electrical charges to communicate between themselves and within the cell, to instruct the cell and body what to do and when.

A simple movement or action requires millions of cells to function in unison to create that movement or action. It then stands to reason that in order for your body to function normally or optimally, it requires the right levels of chemical and hence biochemical reactions in order to do its job.

Ageing or the loss of optimal bodily functioning begins not so much when we reach a certain chronological age, but at such time as our bodily biochemistry is out of balance in greater or lesser amounts over a period of time, causing an array of symptoms from fatigue to other more serious diseases if left unchecked.

Low hormone levels from stress, the absence of important nutrients missing from food, high acidity levels from too much sugar, high pollutant levels and toxicity – in other words an unhealthy biological terrain – does not allow the body to function correctly.

Its natural communication channels and mediums are clouded or blocked. This poor communication ability creates all sorts of problems for the body, stopping it from operating effectively.

It automatically redirects its energy and its immune system in an attempt to rid itself of the excess toxins – pollutants introduced to it through processed and unnatural foods.

In doing so, it lowers its ability to fight viruses and bacterial infections from the surrounding environment.

Cells making up the organs, glands and bones etc. don't divide and renew as they should, in turn making them less efficient and effective and less able to perform their necessary functions, manifesting itself externally into what we see as ageing.

While we are young our bodies (through fewer years of abuse) can adapt to almost anything. That's why young people can go out and play all night, consume large amounts of alcohol and pizza with spicy sausage and wake after a few hours' sleep and put in a full day's work. The down time and recovery for young people are much less, and their bodies can handle more punishment than in the years to follow. But as time goes on we have less and less ability, as our environment slowly deteriorates, to recover and renew.

THE SECRET TO SLOWING YOUR AGEING

To help simplify and summarise the above, the real break-through occurred when scientists discovered that dramatic reductions in the rate at which we age could be achieved by simply altering and rebalancing the state of health of our internal biochemistry, ie. regenerating and rebalancing our levels of hormones, nutrients, vitamins, minerals, enzymes, coenzymes, fats, proteins, sugars, etc. They began to believe and prove that if our biochemical environment is kept healthy and at youthful (optimal) levels, not only will we look and feel years younger but our chances of experiencing the diseases of ageing are far reduced.

Based on this research, the entire goal of **The Anti-ageing Diet** outlined in this book is focused on keeping your internal biochemistry optimal and healthy to allow your body to function at youthful and vibrant levels well beyond your 80th birthday.

YOU ARE WHAT YOU EAT

It has been said you are what you eat!

This revolutionary **Anti-ageing Diet** goes much, much further and deeper than that. It shows that you are not only what you eat, but what you drink, think and do. All these factors combined affect how you age, as all these factors have a direct bearing on the daily state and health of your biochemistry.

Your internal biochemistry is nothing more than the cumulative state (quality and quantity) of your body's entire fluids and chemical profile, including substances such as water, proteins, fats, sugars, hormones, enzymes, coenzymes, minerals, acids and other important substances that allow your body to undertake the critical functions – to grow, detoxify and repair itself on a daily basis.

It is this interaction and the interrelationship between all these substances that determines how well and how effectively your body deals with itself and the billions of chemical actions and reactions that result in keeping you alive and healthy.

CONTROL YOUR AGE FOREVER

Your internal biochemistry is dramatically affected by 5 important factors that you have total control over:

- Stress
- Food you consume
- Exercise or physical exertion
- Pollution and environmental pollutants
- Your daily hormone levels

On a daily basis you have a choice as to what you expose yourself to and what you do. You can choose the foods you eat, the stress you put yourself under (or learn to manage this effectively), the amount of exercise or physical exertion you do, the pollutants and toxins you expose yourself to (for example whether to smoke or not, drink pure water or not etc.), and hence the effect these will all have on your toxicity, acidity, hormones and other internal biochemistry levels.

The point being made is that to succeed in slowing your rate of ageing by following this revolutionary **Anti-ageing**

Diet, your first and most powerful tool is knowledge, and second but equally important is your *Power of Choice*.

To be successful you need to instantly realise you are not a runaway train out of control with regard to your age and health. You have a complete choice over your environment, which in turn has a major bearing on how you age and your long-term health.

Therefore ageing is a matter of choice ... Your choice!

Choose your environment carefully with the help of **The Anti-ageing Diet** and you can by consequence **Choose Your Age**!

Section 2

WHY YOU SHOULD HATE THE WORD DIET!

This might sound strange, considering the title of this book. However, the word 'diet' suggests to the person on a diet that they need to change their eating habits *temporarily*.

To achieve life-long health, longevity, weight loss, usefulness and vitality in advancing years, good looks or for whatever you are interested in **The Anti-ageing Diet** and staying young, **The Anti-ageing Diet** differs dramatically from all the rest in that it is not a quick-fix or short-term diet for weight loss – it is a life-long regime of dedicating yourself to changing the way you conduct your life.

The Anti-ageing Diet will give you much, much more by providing you with cutting-edge knowledge of the foods and other natural practices that are available to you for **life-long peak performance**.

THE FRUSTRATIONS OF DIETING: DIETS SIMPLY DON'T WORK

A 1993 issue of Consumer Reports published in the US put the failure rate for dieters at 75%, and some doctors estimate the failure rate to be as high as 85%.

I attribute much of this to the use of the word 'diet'. A

diet suggests a temporary state of sacrifice in the dieter's mind, but does nothing to educate or address the fundamental or scientific reasons why the dieter is overweight or unhealthy in the first place.

To succeed on diets, dieters need to call on their willpower to give up their 'temporary bad habits' for a period of time to eat foods they dislike or find bland and boring, sacrificing all the good things in life to lose some weight.

If a diet is relying on the basis of good willpower to achieve successful weight loss, it is no wonder the failure rate is so high. No one can go through life continually making sacrifices over the long term.

HOW TO LOSE ALL THE WEIGHT YOU WANT SAFELY AND FOREVER

In order for diets to work (or any long-term change in behaviour, such as quitting smoking, for example) a complete paradigm shift needs to occur, where the dieter or smoker needs to learn to set the right goals, and to have the correct motivation and reasons for dieting or quitting in the first place.

'I want to lose weight' is not a goal. Nor is 'I want to stop smoking' or 'I want to stay young', for that matter.

Successful goal setting requires the author of those goals (you) to set a specific action by a specific time that is realistic and achievable.

Recall the story of the tortoise and the hare. Most dieters want to be the hare, and after abusing themselves and their bodies for so long, want to make it all go away in 5 days or sooner.

What **The Anti-ageing Diet** is asking you to do is relax

when it comes to health. Become more like the tortoise.

Should your goal be to lose weight, you could simply say 'I'm too fat and I'm going on a diet'. But a much better way is to say 'I would like to wear a size X by Christmas' or some other special occasion (whatever date is realistically achievable, given your starting point now). Then you need to work towards your goal – perhaps even by buying an item of clothing in that smaller size now. The proof that this approach works is demonstrated by women planning for their wedding day. Unfortunately, it requires further, permanent goals to be set to maintain health all through your life.

This method of setting achievable goals makes your target more realistic for you and allows you to visualise your end result and provide a time frame in which you can easily achieve it.

This powerful method of goal setting also provides a safety net for you. If you occasionally slip up by eating, drinking or doing something that you shouldn't, you haven't blown your goal completely and you can quickly get back on track.

WHY DIETS DON'T WORK

Diets simply do not work for most people because everybody is different with different needs, wants, tastes and lifestyle.

Our body types are different, our starting points and eating habits are different, our base metabolisms are different, we all have different blood types, our motivations and physiological make up are all different.

All these factors combined make the chances of any one diet (and there have been thousands of them over the years, all claiming to be the ultimate diet) succeeding remote.

HOW TO STAY 30 YEARS OLD FOREVER

Your DNA and genetic make up is completely unique, just like your fingerprints. Only you, among the other 6 billion people on earth, have that specific genetic make up. Therefore, the way you approach your diet, exercise, stress management and nutritional supplementation should also be unique to you.

To successfully read a road map for directions you have to know two things:

1. Where you are now, and
2. Where you want to go.

It is the same when it comes to your **Anti-ageing Diet** and health.

You need to get a realistic fix on where you are now.

To do this you need to get your biomarkers of ageing assessed and recorded.

Biomarkers are biological indicators of your internal biochemistry – measurements such as your cholesterol, homocystene and hormone levels, as well as external markers such as skin elasticity, lung capacity, memory etc.

From this point you will discover with the help of you Anti-ageing specialist where your own deficiencies exist (ie where you are now).

From this information you can begin to set your biomarker ageing goals and what you wish these to be 3, 6 and 9 months from now. These should have values closer to those that indicate optimal health and the internal biochemical profile of a healthy 30-year-old.

According to some of the greatest doctors and scientists in the field of Anti-ageing, it is possible to achieve an optimal biochemical profile of a 30-year-old, no matter what your current chronological age, and maintain this profile until the day you die.

And, yes, you will still die some day, but should you commit to **The Anti-ageing Diet** for the rest of your life, the chances are you will live the majority of your years in sparkling health.

NO ONE IS DYING OF OLD AGE ANYMORE . . .

In this modern age, we are dying of nutritional deficiencies and man-made plagues such as heart disease, cancer and diabetes. Not many people today die of old age. The 3 leading causes of death (based on US data) are:

- 1899 – influenza, diarrhoea, pneumonia
- 1999 – heart disease, cancer, stroke
- 2046 – suicide, homicide, aerospace accidents.

YOUR OWN PERSONALISED ANTI-AGEING DIET

It is important to remember you are a unique individual.

You age in a different way and at a different rate to any other person. This illustrates the importance of having an **Anti-ageing Diet** that is specifically designed to address your needs. In fact, indiscriminate use of Anti-ageing food, products and treatments may not be helpful, and could even be harmful to your health.

This step is the most important aspect to Anti-ageing, because without comprehensive knowledge and testing of each individual, and proper prescriptions, any diet could either be wasted or, worse, dangerous to your health.

Even though **Anti-ageing Diets** use all-natural substances such as foods, vitamins, minerals, herbs and amino acids, as well as hormone-balancing therapies, it is important to consume these substances in exactly the right amounts for your individual biochemistry.

WHY THE ANTI-AGEING DIET IS THE ULTIMATE DIET AND WORKS SO WELL

The Anti-ageing Diet is not like any diet you have seen or heard of before, and I am sure you have seen or been exposed to many, with varying degrees of success. It's not about counting calories or denying yourself the 'good things' in life.

It's about understanding how the body works and working with it naturally to get yourself to a state of optimal health all through your life.

If your body is in optimal health, it will naturally regulate its own weight, keep your skin and other organs well preserved to keep you functioning well and looking young, as well as fight off viruses and diseases with a strong and powerful immune system that is in good working order.

The Anti-ageing Diet is far, far more than just the latest fad or weight-loss program. It is the ultimate life-long diet, exercise and body-maintenance program that will last (more than an expected lifetime) for most.

Most people today are unwittingly eating and drinking themselves to a slow and painful death, or at least to a life far shorter and of lower quality than they would like or is possible.

With the powerful life-changing knowledge you will gain through reading and understanding this book, I guarantee you will never need another eating plan, weight-loss or liver-cleansing diet again.

Section 3

SO WHAT IS THE ANTI-AGEING DIET?

No matter what your genetic blueprint, **The Anti-ageing Diet** will help you live a longer, healthier, more fulfilling life, by educating and informing you on a safe, natural way to peak performance.

The Anti-ageing Diet covers 5 main area that you can take control of to influence your life, not through a short-term 'diet' but through sensible, life-long daily choices and habits.

The 5 essential areas making up **The Anti-ageing Diet** are the practical applications and tools used by Anti-ageing specialists to combat the causes of ageing outlined in an earlier section.

These are:

Major Causes of Ageing	Anti-ageing Diet	Tools
Stress	Stress Management	Meditation, Exercise
Poor Nutrition	Nutritional Balancing	Change your diet and nutritional supplementation
Lack of Exercise	Correct Exercise Program	Regular exercise

Pollutants and Toxins	Detoxification	Lymphatic Drainage, Avoidance techniques, antioxidants
Hormone Deficiencies	Hormone Re-balancing	Exercise and hormone boosters and supplements

THE SECRET TO STAYING YOUNG

Many of the tools used in **The Anti-ageing Diet** just listed above work because they combine to increase and rebalance the internal biochemistry, natural hormone levels and pH levels in the body.

Our lifestyles today, especially our poor diet, exercise, and stress regime take a heavy toll on our bodies after years of unknowing abuse. Most people in western society today are living in a dangerous zone, on unbalanced biological terrain. This could be compared to a time bomb, ready to explode at any minute, when it comes to their health.

Mental stress, pollution, poor nutrition and lack of exercise all contribute towards massive toxicity and chemical impurities and imbalances. This cumulatively causes the body to labour and struggle to perform its daily functions. What we see as a result of this is people living with low energy levels, fatigue, more stress, poor health, regular sickness and the onset of life-threatening disease.

Left unchecked, this will cause many people to live a poorer quality of life and be faced with the possibility of disease affecting one or more of their organs, such as heart disease, cancer, stroke, Alzheimer's, Parkinson's, osteoporosis, diabetes etc.

EARLY-WARNING SYSTEM TO AGEING

In order to limit our risk of contracting these diseases of 'affluence', we must not wait until we show outward manifestations of sickness, which in some cases may be too late. We must realise we have an early-warning system – our biological terrain – and address our internal biochemistry by re-balancing our hormones, nutrients, minerals and pH levels, as well as aiming to reduce or manage our daily stress.

Anti-ageing medicine has shown that no one living in western society is immune to these imbalances.

Modern farming practices producing the food we consume in all its forms have severely altered the nutritional value of what we eat. Not only have we lost up to 90% of the traditional value of food through farming and then pro-cessing, we are also consuming large quantities of herbicides, pesticides, industrial chemicals and artificial hormones that have crept into our food chain.

These unnatural substances in small quantities are not toxic enough to cause instant disability or death, but over the years they accumulate in our bodies and take an ever-increasing toll on our ability to fight off the effects of ageing and disease.

The goal of Anti-ageing specialists is to provide optimum nutrition to the body, as well as reverse the effects of years of damage, by re-stimulating, and in some cases supple-menting, hormones to optimal levels, and help our bodies remove toxic waste build-up.

The body functions correctly through a complex inter-action between the cells, their DNA and the brain. Hormones and enzymes are effectively the messengers between these components.

In order for the body to function in its millions of daily activities, our hormone levels need to be undisturbed. For most of us, this is not the case. We suffer from an imbalance of many Anti-ageing hormones such as HGH (human growth hormone), DHEA (dehydroxiandrestonenine), melatonin, testosterone, progesterone and oestrogen, to name just a few.

FOOD ON THE ANTI-AGEING DIET

FOODS THAT KEEP YOU YOUNG

There is no doubt the food we eat on a daily basis will make an enormous difference to our lives and how fast we age.

Of all the topics covered in this book there is no doubt food is the most emotionally charged, because for most of us food is much more than a source of nutrition. It is a source of comfort, a symbol of love, a recreational past time, a social event and even a form of entertainment.

Most people don't actually believe their diets are that bad. In truth, they may be terrible, but it's all a matter of perspective and education.

Having a piece of chocolate or a hamburger will not kill you, but if you make a lifetime habit of eating these perhaps they will.

Most people today are unwittingly eating and drinking themselves to a slow and painful death, or at least to a life far shorter and of lower quality than they would like or which is possible.

We are heavily influenced in what we eat by our parents, our friends and the millions of dollars spent on marketing and advertising, bombarding us with mixed messages consciously and subliminally shaping our choices and behaviour.

Our lifestyle make us time-poor, while greater disposable incomes entice us to spend less time preparing our own meals and offer us more and more opportunities to buy fast, prepared or processed food.

Who has the time today to grow their own vegetables or grind their own flour and bake bread? More and more meals today are eaten outside the home or prepared by someone else. **The Anti-ageing Diet** eating strategy will give you some important guidelines and principles to follow.

Following **The Anti-ageing Diet** guidelines to eating is not scary, nor will it deprive you of the good things in life.

In fact, the basis of the food you consume on your **Anti-ageing Diet** is about discovering for yourself the foods that you really enjoy but which are also healthy for you, and eating less of the things that will put strain on your body and cut your health span short, accelerating your ageing.

As far as **The Anti-ageing Diet** is concerned, everything you eat and do either accelerates your ageing or works to slow it down. It is our intention in this book to make you aware of what these things are.

While **The Anti-ageing Diet** includes food in its prescription to slowing your ageing it also understand the interaction with other ageing factors we have covered in this book.

ONE GREAT REASON WHY DIETS DON'T WORK

The great flaw of all other diets is that they work on the premise that what is good for the goose is good for the gander. This is not the case, and this is the exact reason why so many diets don't work or fail to produce any significant result.

Every person is unique and has different genes. Therefore, no two people will behave in the same biological way.

Dr Peter D'Adamo, in his book *Eat Right Diet*, for the first time makes this point very well. His theory for the basis of a great diet is your blood type.

He explains this by pointing out that all blood is not the same. That is why only certain blood-type donors are used to supply blood to certain blood-type recipients. The body will reject the wrong type of blood.

This is old news in medicine. The reason this occurs is because each blood type has different antigens or chemical markers which help the body discriminate between foreign friendly substances.

If a substance entering the body through the skin or digestive system is, for example, identified as a foreign invader by the mismatch of antigens, it sets off a chemical reaction of the immune system to search for and destroy those substances.

Through numerous years of research and experimentation, Dr D'Adamo identified that different foods contain a substance called lectins.

When you eat a food that has lectins that are incompatible with your blood-type antigen, your body reacts to these food substances in way similar to the way the body reacts to a viral or bacterial infection.

As a result of this, many foods that your mother, father, friend or sister eat that may be beneficial (or harmful) to them, may be harmful (or beneficial) to you.

The difference is the blood type.

WHY HARMFUL FOODS AGE
YOU FAST

Therefore, instead of your body's immune system fighting disease and infection as it was designed to do, it spends most of its time and reserves fighting the incompatible food you are eating. Over a period of time this weakens your immune system, causing your body to rapidly age and deteriorate into ill health.

If you stop for a moment and consider this logic, it makes perfect sense.

Dr D'Adamo has published a comprehensive list of what foods are good, neutral or bad for each blood type in his book, or these can be provided to you at your Anti-ageing centre.

TO STAY AND LOOK YOUNG EAT
MORE FAT

Ask yourself . . . why is it that with all the hype and promotion about eating high-carbohydrate, low-fat diets, with the abundance of low-fat foods on the market and the popularity of health clubs and personal trainers, more and more people are obese or overweight than ever before?

In the current focus on low-fat foods and the dangers of cholesterol, it is important to remember that the body needs a certain amount of some kinds of fat.

Natural fats provide the body with a concentrated form of energy and allow vitamins such as A and E to be digested. Fats are also used by the body to maintain cellular structure.

So, it is essential that we do eat fat in our diet. Fats, however, come in two forms – saturated (bad fat) from animals and unsaturated (good fats) from vegetables and fish oils.

Saturated fats are the worst type of fat you can eat because these fats increase your LDL cholesterol levels.

Unsaturated fats comes in two categories – poly-unsaturated or mono-unsaturated, referring to the length of the fatty acid molecule, poly-unsaturated being a long chain of fatty acid molecules and mono-unsaturated being a short chain.

Unsaturated oils such as olive oil, flaxseeds oil, evening primrose oil and cod liver oil are the best fats to consume. They actually lower LDL cholesterol and raise HDL cholesterol.

These are called **Omega 3** and **Omega 6** essential fatty acids and are particularly important in helping prevent heart disease, arthritis and cancer and for a young and healthy-looking skin.

These fats are called essential fatty acids because the body cannot produce them and they need to be consumed daily as part of your **Anti-ageing Diet**.

Suggested Anti-ageing doses Omega 3 and 6 – 1000mg per day.

HOW TO EAT THE RIGHT FAT

When eating fats, it is best to eat them unheated or cooked as heating or cooking changes their composition and removes the beneficial aspects for proper nutrition. Cold-pressed oils, such as cold-pressed olive oil, are your best source of good fats.

Therefore do not feel that you are doing the right thing by frying your children chips in olive oil as opposed to any other oil you may use. Heating fat or buying fats/oils that have been heated is not the way to go.

Don't be fooled by margarine marketing. Margarine is

modified fat that has been hydrogenised, ie. converted from a liquid to a solid.

It raises your blood cholesterol level, even though it contains less cholesterol than butter.

It is better to eat butter if you must, but best not to have either. The same applies to any other food product claiming to be low in cholesterol. If it has been cooked in oil or fat it will raise your own LDL cholesterol levels.

Another very important point to be made is about the body's metabolism of fats. Fats are a concentrated form of energy, and the body requires that energy to perform its daily functions. However, because it needs to unlock the energy from fat before it can be used, it will first use the sugar in the blood, then the sugar stored in the muscles before it begins converting the fats in the blood stream and lastly the fat stored in the fat cells (it is these cells that makes us look fat) for energy. (More in the next chapter)

What this means, is that if you are consuming too much sugary or high-glycaemic-index carbohydrates (complex sugars that are easily converted to sugar), for example refined flour found in breads, pastas or starchy foods such as potatoes (see attached list), and also eating too much fat regardless of whether it is saturated or unsaturated, your body will not use it and simply store it as fat.

FATS AND SUGARS JUST DON'T MIX

If you are going to eat any form of carbohydrate, especially refined/processed carbohydrates, in a meal, it's best not to combine that with fats of any kind.

Many of the things we have been brought up on as kids

fall into this category, such as cheese sandwiches, macaroni and cheese, bread and butter (or margarine) or even worse bread, butter and jam. It is these habits we develop as kids that make it difficult to give up later in life when they do us the most damage.

When you do eat fat, it's best to eat it in the absence of any refined carbohydrates or sugar and eat fat with a protein food or with unprocessed food such as salad and vegetables. If this rule is not followed you will find it increasingly difficult to maintain a healthy weight and cholesterol level throughout your life.

Eating more fat and less carbohydrate is healthy for you, as long as this is balanced with the right protein level. These balances vary from individual to individual depending on your age, genes, starting point (current level of body fat) and level of physical activity.

Eating more of the good fat and less refined carbohydrates also teaches your body to use this as a fuel source and not to immediately store it. It will not do this, however, if there is too much insulin present in the blood.

Insulin again is released due to the excess consumption of high-glycaemic-index foods – foods that are easily absorbed from the stomach and quickly converted to blood sugar eg alcohol, sugar, any foods high in sugars, most refined carbohydrates such as white pasta, white rice, desserts, ice creams, chocolates etc.

That is why manufactured products such as commercial chocolate cause weight gains. There is no real nutritional value in these foods, yet they are high in both fats and sugars, sugars causing the body to raise its insulin level when entering the blood, which in turn stores the fat provided at the same time by the chocolate.

BEWARE: NOT ALL CARBOHYDRATES ARE THE SAME

You will find people who are on high-carbohydrate diets, especially those who consume high-glycaemic-index foods, even if they do exercise always seem to be hungry and easily put on fat. The reason this occurs is that high-glycaemic-index carbohydrates enter the body as sugar very quickly. This raises the level of insulin secreted and any excess calories that are not immediately required are converted and stored as fat.

Now, although the total calories consumed for the daily requirement may be sufficient, the excess calories that have just been consumed are removed from the blood and stored, dropping the blood sugar levels (hypoglycaemia), triggering hunger and a search for more food, which usually consists of more high-glycaemic-index food – and the cycle goes on.

Fat gain is made even worse if these carbohydrates are consumed together with fats.

TEACH YOUR BODY TO BURN FAT, NOT SUGAR

By eating more *good* fat as part of your balanced **Anti-ageing Diet** and less high-glycaemic-index carbohydrates, your body will produce less insulin and begin to rely on converting and using fat as an energy source.

Because we are eating too many carbohydrates and have not taught our bodies to burn fat (in fact we have done the opposite: made our bodies believe we are in famine times and that fat should be stored) we become hungry again shortly after eating the refined carbohydrates.

Our bodies quickly use up the sugar in the blood and muscles, and because they are inefficient at using the energy we have stored as excess fat hunger results.

By eating more good fats, the body begins to realise there is no shortage of food, we are not in famine times and it will use the fat readily. But this re-education of the body to burn fat takes time.

This may explain why many people on a high-carbohydrate, low-fat diet who do regular exercise still have difficulty losing weight.

We will cover this in a later chapter, however, when you do exercise, especially high-intensity exercise such as aerobics, swimming or running, your body is using blood sugar as its energy source before it burns fat. Fat-burning only kicks in once these sugar stores are depleted

This is why after intensive exercise of between 40–60 minutes, people get that 'starving' feeling. This makes them want to restore their blood sugars quickly and they generally crave the refined (high-glycaemic-index) carbohydrates to try to quickly replace the low blood sugar levels. This error in exercise and food selection simply increases the blood sugar levels and causes the body to deposit the excess calories as fat, causing the exercise to have little or no effect in helping reduce weight or fat.

Beside the immediate fat concerns, eating too many carbohydrates as we discussed raises insulin levels at each meal.

Insulin is the hormone that is responsible for triggering the transport of sugar into the cell. As time goes by, especially if there is too much insulin present all the time, our cells may become more and more insulin resistant, requiring more insulin each time to get the energy the cell needs. This process over a period of time increases the risk of insulin-resistant diabetes in adults, which is a major cause of many different illnesses and death.

STILL CONFUSED ABOUT CHOLESTEROL?

Cholesterol still remains very confusing to most people. What most people don't know is that 90% of our cholesterol is manufactured by our own body. Many factors increase your cholesterol production – smoking, high blood pressure, liver problems exacerbated by a diet high in toxic additives and preservatives, inadequate exercise, too much body fat, stress, depression. Consuming too much fat does not necessarily convert to cholesterol, but tends to aggravate these other factors and will indirectly raise your cholesterol level.

Cholesterol travels through the body and is needed to make bile, hormones and vitamin D. The cells take what they need and the rest is left in the blood stream. The body can only use HDL cholesterol obtained through plants and vegetable products, and not LDL cholesterol obtained through animal products. Therefore, LDL cholesterol usually ends up as plaque that clogs our artery walls.

FIBRE: A GREAT ANTI-AGEING TOOL

We've heard much about high fibre in our diets over the past few years. Much of it is true. A high-fibre diet tends to soak up fat and is essential to a healthy digestive system. It helps us avoid many age-related diseases, such as bowel cancer, gall stones, diabetes, colitis, haemorrhoids, hernia and varicose veins.

PROTEIN: HOW MUCH SHOULD YOU EAT?

Too much protein is bad for you, as is too little, but how much is right for you?

This answer depends on many things – your age, your level of physical activity, your lean body weight, your level of stress etc.

Too much protein puts an unwarranted strain on your digestive and elimination systems and it causes your body's pH balance to become too acidic, reducing the effectiveness of your immune system and hormones. On the other hand, too little protein will inhibit muscle, hair, skin and cell growth and repair.

Either way, too much or too little protein will accelerate ageing and possible disease.

Finding the right balance is important for you, and this begins with a consultation with an experienced Anti-ageing nutritionist.

Depending on your blood type and other factors, your protein can come from a number of sources. The sources recommended on your **Anti-ageing Diet**, however, are beans, grains and legumes, supplemented with fish and low-fat dairy. These are far superior in slowing ageing than red meat or chicken.

IS SALT REALLY BAD FOR YOU?

It's not the salt you add to your food that's the problem. It's the salt that's already in there that could be.

Salt is so widely used in cooking that unless you cook all your own food from fresh, natural sources, you are being exposed to high levels of salt without realising it.

Read the labels of most pre-prepared or processed food and you will verify this. Salt ends up in the most unlikely places – gravies, peanut butter, salad dressing, canned fish, cheese, processed meats, smoked food products, frozen dinners, potato chips, popcorn, canned vegetables, condiments and sauces, soups and meat tenderisers.

If you do need to add a little salt be mindful of what's already in you food before you pick up the salt shaker.

Many people find success in substituting other herbs including basil, red pepper or lemon. Others have discovered that, after a few weeks on what seems like a bland no-salt diet, suddenly foods take on a whole new range of flavours and the palate adjusts and rejects the salty taste it used to crave.

SO SWEET YET SO DEADLY

We discussed high-glycaemic-index carbohydrates above. Sugar is the worst kind. It is terribly bad for you. Whether you are consuming it from a sugar jar, or as raw sugar, honey, glucose, dextrose, corn syrup or many other hidden sources, it puts enormous strain on your biological terrain.

People with a sweet tooth suffer from a yo-yo condition of hypoglycaemia (low blood sugar). They crave something sweet to give them energy. Soon after eating it they get a short energy hit, but then come crashing down as insulin kicks in to try to normalise the levels, followed by more sugar cravings to bring energy levels up again.

These people often experience frequent fatigue, trembling, rapid heart beat, lack of concentration, memory problems and emotional instability.

Sugar addicts who drink caffeine in coffee or cola drinks experience a double rush and double crash. Ironically, the very substance that picks you up is the one that drains you, so that you are caught in this vicious cycle of needing coffee or sugar to wake you up and keep you going.

Breaking this cycle altogether will prolong your life and give you back your sustained energy. Again, most sugar consumed is hidden in processed foods and as a result we are unknowingly eating far too much sugar.

It is imperative for you to cut down your sugar consumption on your **Anti-ageing Diet**. You will not even miss this extra sugar once you become aware of it and substitute foods that contain no sugar that you still enjoy, like fresh unprocessed foods.

Read the labels of the foods you eat to become aware of just how much sugar you are eating.

Beware: manufacturers try to disguise this by breaking up sugar counts by listing sugar as dextrose, corn syrup and other forms of sweeteners to make the amount of sugar look less significant.

Section 5

NUTRITION ON THE ANTI-AGEING DIET
by John Gearon

WHY WE ARE EATING LESS FAT BUT WE ARE GETTING FATTER

For the past 10–15 years we have been consistently focusing on low–fat foods, reduced–fat foods and non–fat foods. On an average percentage basis, we are getting fatter and fatter. The interesting thing of late is that a lot of the anti–cellulite treatments that are on the market actually have between 45 and 65% essential fats.

Think about it. We are putting less fats in our diet, in the way of saturated and unsaturated fats and all other fats that are hidden in foods, yet overall we are consistently getting fatter. Is it the fats in our diets that are making us fatter? No, it isn't. We have had a good look at this on **The Anti-ageing Diet** and we have designed a whole new food pyramid to move away from this trend.

THE NEW NUTRITIONAL PYRAMID – A HEALTH BREAKTHROUGH

To appreciate the new pyramid we have to actually look at the old dietary guidelines we have been focusing on for the past 20–30 years. The five-food-group pyramid that has been used as a benchmark by dietitians, nutritionists, anti-cancer foundations, heart foundations, food companies etc looks like this:

12345 + FOOD & NUTRITIONAL PLAN★

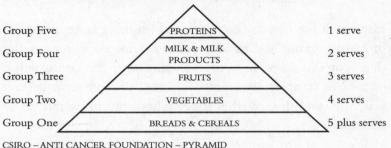

Group Five	PROTEINS	1 serve
Group Four	MILK & MILK PRODUCTS	2 serves
Group Three	FRUITS	3 serves
Group Two	VEGETABLES	4 serves
Group One	BREADS & CEREALS	5 plus serves

CSIRO – ANTI CANCER FOUNDATION – PYRAMID

One of the major contributing factors to why we are getting fatter is this old food pyramid. The bottom line is 5+ serves of breads and cereals (refined carbohydrates). Most people assume that 5+ means endless/unlimited, so they have a large serving of pasta, cereals or breads and only count the calories in the sauces.

INDUSTRIAL AGEING

The bottom line of Group One refined carbohydrates of the food pyramid has been around only since the industrial age. The industrial age gave us technology to manufacture and store breads, grains cereals and pastas. Prior to the industrial age, the food pyramid of hundreds of years ago would have been mostly made up of vegetables, fruit and meat options. Since the industrial age came about we have inserted the largest food group on the bottom line of the pyramid – refined-carbohydrate breads and cereals. This is one of the main reasons why people all over the world are getting fatter and unhealthier.

HOW CARBOHYDRATES CREPT INTO OUR DIETS

History shows that the concept of consuming large quantities of cereals, grains and carbohydrates originated from societies that required large amounts of manpower for construction of ancient temples, pyramids and other massive structures. It was the wealthy of the time who commissioned these structures.

Wealth at the time was determined by the amount of land, gold or livestock one possessed. The proposition of feeding livestock (protein) to this massive workforce was inconceivable. Thus grain which was in abundance and used to fatten livestock also became the primary food in the workers' diet.

Studies have found that these workers and slaves who were working long hours performing heavy labour and expending massive amounts of calories managed to maintain a higher body fat percentage than that of the wealthy who traditionally performed minimal activity.

The reason is that the grains used to fatten livestock also fatten humans. The grains have a high-glycaemic reaction that produces excess quantities of insulin. Excess insulin is explained in detail in other sections.

WHY LOW-FAT, HIGH-CARBOHYDRATE, LOW-PROTEIN DIETS DON'T WORK

One of the other reasons why low-fat, high-carbohydrate diets don't work is they do not make distinctions between the two groups of carbohydrates.

1. Complex – vegetables & fruits.
2. Refined – cereals, beards and grains.

Each also contains two types of carbohydrates, low glycaemic and high glycaemic. Low-glycaemic carbohydrates are absorbed slowly in the system and do not cause a rapid rise in blood sugar. High-glycaemic carbohydrates, on the other hand, are quickly absorbed and cause a rapid rise in blood sugar. This is important because when you have a rapid rise in blood sugar it causes an insulin reaction – a large burst of insulin into the blood stream. Insulin then removes excessive glycogen and blood sugar from the blood and stores it in the muscle cells. Any excess glycogen (blood sugar) is converted to fat/triglycerides, for storage in the fat/adipose cells of the body, around your tummy, hips and thighs. Therefore, eating a high-glycaemic food causes your body to store carbohydrates as fat and not expel energy. This is why most low-fat, high-carbohydrates diets fail, even though they are keeping calories to a minimum.

SUCCESS ON HIGH-PROTEIN, LOW-CARBOHYDRATE DIETS

For the body to expend energy it will source it first from

the blood and muscle sugars. Once that is depleted it will burn fat stores for fuel. Maintaining diet intake of high protein and low-glycaemic carbohydrates will greatly reduce the blood sugar and insulin levels and increase the fat stores to be burnt as fuel.

HIGH-REFINED-CARBOHYDRATE DIETS

Another reason why a high-carbohydrate diet doesn't work is because when increasing the percentage of carbohydrates in their diet, most people focus on increasing their intake of refined carbohydrates – breads and cereals – and not complex carbohydrates such as fresh fruits and vegetables.

It is easier to get refined carbohydrates than go to a fresh fruit and vegetable shop. Fresh fruit and vegetable shops used to be in abundance, around every corner. Now, in their place are fast food and bread chains. When dieting, the water content of the foods you consume should be around 70%. High-refined-carbohydrate foods have next to zero water content. You can understand how this affects your success on a high-refined-carbohydrate diet.

THE BREAD STORY

Most people don't appreciate what we do to bread, or actually realise it has now become one of the major components of modern diets.

You have to look at what we do to the simple grain. The wheat grain is ground into flour. We then add liquid, yeast and preservatives along with many other additives to form dough. After kneading, the dough is put into a high-temperature oven, whereby the whole molecular structure of the grain is altered by the heat, which dries it out and destroys any vitamin or mineral content. The heat changes the configuration and raises the glycaemic levels, because the dough is baked to form a hard, firm crust. The dough has now become a loaf of bread with its hard, crusty shell keeping any moisture that may be left trapped inside. The preservatives are added to increase shelf life.

The loaf of bread then has a slice of bread cut from it, exposing any moisture that may have been trapped. The slice is placed in a toaster, the temperature is turned up to dry it out even more and the molecular structure changes once again.

We heat it, carbonise it, blacken it, and char it to the point we now call it toast. The toast is then spread with some saturated fats (butter, margarine or cheese) then usually spread some more with totally high-glycaemic carbohydrates (sugar jams or fruit spreads).

We then eat it and expect our body to attempt to digest it! The only thing this item called toast really has left in it is some insoluble fibre and high-glycaemic carbohydrates that will raise your insulin level.

Because it is so dry, it is harsh on our digestive system. I'm sure you can now understand why we feel bloated after having too much bread.

LOOKING AT WHEAT

Most refined-carbohydrate food sources are composed of wheat.

Most wheat products cause a very high glycaemic reaction to the system. They also produce allergic reactions in our system with a wide degree of symptomology

The interesting thing is that if people put their hand in a bag of wheat and then pulled it out, most would find that their arm is very itchy and scratchy from the allergic reaction to the wheat grains. The skin is a more durable organ than our internal digestive tract. We never for a moment think that the bloating, the distension or the irritable bowel syndromes we are getting is caused by these wheat products.

We just put it down to everything else.

POTATOES – THE FOOD WE WERE NEVER MEANT TO EAT

It is time to look at the simple potato, which has become a popular and convenient part of our staple diets.

How and why did this happen when we know it to be one of the major contributing factors to our ever-increasing waist lines?

We all know that if a potato is green it is toxic, as it is when it is sprouting. There is only a small window of time in which we can safely prepare a potato for consumption. We would never eat a potato raw because it is indigestible, tastes horrible and our body would react violently to it.

So what do we do ... we boil, steam, fry or bake it for anything from 5-45 minutes, to get enough heat or moisture in it so it is palatable enough to eat. It still has little taste, unless we saturated it with fat, so we proceed to add butter, salt and lots of other additives to get it to a semi-edible state.

After all this preparation, we have added so much fat to it, that the amount of calories of cooked fat is higher than the calories from the potato.

Think about this next time you eat a potato.

Where did the potato originate from? The Irish had an

abundance of them during the great Depression, simply because the animals would not eat them and people had never really wanted to. Animals are a lot smarter than we give them credit for. They instinctively know not to eat a raw potato, yet we, the smarter species, have devised a way to disguise the potato to the extent that we can now allow ourselves to enjoy it, because it tastes like something else . . . Who are we fooling? Certainly not our bodies.

We hear about this new frontier of genetic engineering and we get worried about it, yet we've been doing it in our kitchens for years. We daily use 'kitchen engineering' to successfully modify our foods and to slowly kill ourselves.

We have always known that potato starches are used in the form of adhesives, for wallpaper glue, stick glues, children's glues etc. Do you really want to start eating a vegetable that is also used as glue? Ask yourself what must this be doing to your digestive system on the inside?

To speed up our metabolism and slow ageing we must avoid this type of vegetable starch, along with some of the other refined-carbohydrate starches being put into our digestive system. A major point to remember is that eating heavy starches has a dehydrating effect on our body as water is needed to break these down. In addition, high-glycaemic-index starches such as potatoes also cause a rapid rise in our insulin levels that will convert any excess calories into fat, which is what we are trying to avoid.

MILK: A POOR SUBSTITUTE

Ask yourself this question? Would you actually go and lie down under a cow and start sucking its nipple. The answer would be 'no', but that's exactly what we do each day when we drink our milk. And if that's not bad enough, we don't just drink it as milk, we take it, process it, pasteurise it, put colour in it, put flavour in it and call it flavoured (mucus) milk or cappuccino.

Humans are the only species that continues to drink milk-based products after they have been weaned off them as infants.

There is a lot of conjecture regarding the mucous-producing properties of milk and milk-related products in our digestive system. Lactose intolerance is creeping more and more into our vocabulary every day.

There is great Anti-ageing benefit in using any one of the many milk-substitute products currently on the market, products that are fortified with calcium, lactobacillus and phytoestrogens.

They offer all the benefits of cows' milk without the health-related concerns. For conditions such as eczema, asthma and runny noses, one of the first things the allergists remove from the diet is milk.

So, why are nutritionists and dietitians educating parents to persist in the use of milk products? If a milk product has an allergic reaction on a child, you can be certain as an adult the same reaction would be present. We lose the ability to break down and digest milk effectively shortly after we stop breastfeeding.

However, adults who continue to consume milk over many years have had their systems so beaten up by milk products and other everyday foods, that their level of dramatic reaction to milk is quite limited because their immune system has been so suppressed against it.

A REVOLUTIONARY BREAKTHROUGH: THE NEW FOOD PYRAMID THAT WILL KEEP YOU YOUNG

The new food pyramid that we have designed on **The Anti-ageing Diet** is based on longevity, peak performance and optimum health.

There are four food groups to the inverted pyramid. The major focus on the largest section at the top is 40–35% low-glycaemic fresh vegetables and fresh fruits (this does not include all fruit and vegetables).

Our second-largest area is 30–25% protein, focusing on fresh fish, red and white meats, soy products and beans and legumes.

The third section, 15–20%, should be refined carbohydrates, but only from low-glycaemic sources. The bottom section, 15–20%, is essential fats.

ACID VERSUS ALKALINE FOODS

The human body functions most optimally when in an acid/alkaline balanced state.

Our biochemical reactions work best in a slightly alkaline biological terrain (blood, urine and saliva). Human blood pH ranges from 7.35 to 7.4 pH. The ranges are acid 0pH, alkaline 14 pH and neutral 7pH.

When fat is used for energy instead of carbohydrates, an acid residue is produced that causes a rise in your body's pH levels. Most methods of reducing fat stores create an increase of acidic residue.

This leads to the feelings of discomfort, irritability,

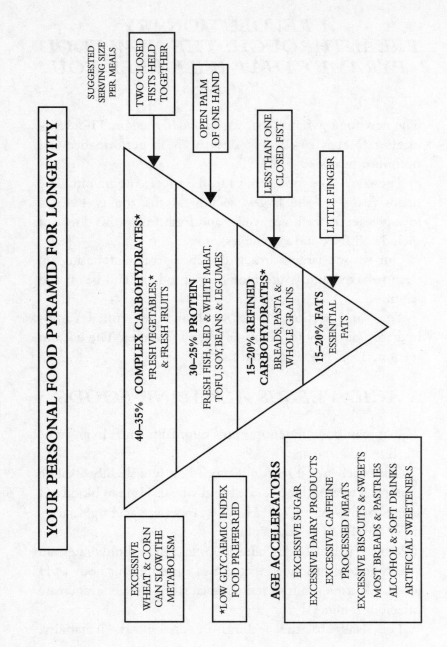

YOUR PERSONAL FOOD PYRAMID FOR LONGEVITY

SUGGESTED SERVING SIZE PER MEALS

40–35% COMPLEX CARBOHYDRATES*
FRESH VEGETABLES,*
& FRESH FRUITS

TWO CLOSED FISTS HELD TOGETHER

30–25% PROTEIN
FRESH FISH, RED & WHITE MEAT,
TOFU, SOY, BEANS & LEGUMES

OPEN PALM OF ONE HAND

15–20% REFINED CARBOHYDRATES*
BREADS, PASTA &
WHOLE GRAINS

LESS THAN ONE CLOSED FIST

15–20% FATS
ESSENTIAL FATS

LITTLE FINGER

EXCESSIVE WHEAT & CORN CAN SLOW THE METABOLISM

*LOW GLYCAEMIC INDEX FOOD PREFERRED

AGE ACCELERATORS

EXCESSIVE SUGAR
EXCESSIVE DAIRY PRODUCTS
EXCESSIVE CAFFEINE
PROCESSED MEATS
EXCESSIVE BISCUITS & SWEETS
MOST BREADS & PASTRIES
ALCOHOL & SOFT DRINKS
ARTIFICIAL SWEETENERS

headache, nausea, upset stomach, and fatigue. These negative reactions make it very difficult for individuals to stick to a fat-reducing program.

Low-glycaemic carbohydrates and other low-acid foods will assist in further reducing body pH imbalances. Dark green vegetables are an excellent source to increase the alkaline content of your biological terrain, which will reduce the acid effects of burning fat stores.

THOUSAND-YEAR-OLD FATS

History has shown our ancestors ate a diet consisting of lean meats, fresh fish and large amounts of fresh fruits, raw vegetables, seeds and nuts.

This diet had a balance of essential fatty acids (EFA), Omega-6 and Omega-3. Our current diet, however, has changed this natural balance because the industrial process has removed the majority of Omega-3 fats from our foods.

EFAs have different molecular structures than the saturated fats which can cause us harm.

Essential fatty acids (EFA), Omega-6 and Omega-3 may help to increase our energy levels, while reducing blood pressure, level of triglycerides and blood cholesterol. Cholesterol has been blamed for heart disease, but recent studies have shown that high cholesterol levels in some cases can be attributed to symptom deficiencies of EFA.

To reduce your chances of becoming deficient in essential fatty acids, we recommend on your **Anti-ageing Diet** that you eat more natural foods in their unprocessed state. This works best for reducing the risk of cardiovascular disease, but it will also assist in preventing other diseases of ageing.

A low-fat food selection can be healthy, but only when

it includes eating foods that are low in saturated fat and high in balanced EFAs. Raw green vegetables, fresh fish, seed and flaxseed oil are a rich source of essential fatty acids.

JUICING VEGETABLES OR FRUITS

We get asked a lot 'can we juice our fruits'? The response generally is to say yes, fine, by all means juice away – if you have to – but throw away the juice and eat the pulp.

The pulp that is separated in the juicer has all of the fibre plus a lot of the nutrients, vitamins and minerals. What you are discarding is what is most beneficial.

The pulp is going to stop you from having a high-glycaemic reaction to the high concentration of sugars that occur from juicing fruit. Once again it is back to that insulin overload and your body actually transferring all of that excess sugar into triglycerides and storing it as fat.

When you juice for a normal glass you need 4–6 pieces of fruit and end up with a high concentration of calories. You will also find that you are going to have a high sugar reaction and still be hungry. This is because your insulin levels accelerate and are quite high from the sugar concentration.

There is a solution.

If you need to drink your fruit or vegetables use a powerful blender that purees the fruits and vegetables to a drinkable pulp.

You will not only have fewer calories, but you will also have a lower glycaemic reaction within your system and feel more fulfilled. Your need to have more and more fruit and vegetables is maximised and you are having fewer calories. And because you will be experiencing less of an insulin rush you will be storing less sugars as fats.

Overall, fruits are always better eaten whole. The next best option is to blend them in a powerful blender that will pulp and not discard any of the contents. Note: Keeping fruits and vegetables separate will optimise the nutritional health benefits because you are not mixing together the alkaline (vegetables) and acids (some high sugar fruits).

GLYCAEMIC FOODS INDEX FOR PEAK PERFORMANCE

LOW-GLYCAEMIC INDEX
Less than 50

Most green vegetables		**CEREAL GRAINS**	
Leafy Vegetables		Barley, pearled	36
Broccoli		Rye Kernels	47
Spinach			
		LEGUMES	
FRUIT		Dhal, Bengal lentils	12
Plum	25	Peanuts	15
Grapefruit	26	Soybeans, dried	20
Peach	29	Soybeans, canned	22
Pear	34	Black-eyed peas	33
Apple juice	45	Lentils, green, dried	33
Grape	45	Lima beans	36
Pineapple – Canned		Navy beans	40
Unsweetened	48	Kidney beans, dried	43
Apple	49	Butter beans	46
		Chickpeas, dried	47
BREADS		Peas, dried	49
Rye, whole grain	42		
Barley, coarse, scalded kernels	48	**SUGARS**	
		Fructose	25
BREAKFAST CEREALS			
Bran	31		
Oats Rolled, long cooking	49		

INTERMEDIATE-GLYCAEMIC INDEX
50 to 75

VEGETABLES

Sweet potato	59
Yam	62
Beet	64

FRUIT

Orange	56
Banana, green	56
Orange juice	65
Pineapple	66

BREADS

Barley, coarse	57
Rye, pumpernickel	68
Wheat, coarse	73

BREAKFAST CEREALS

White, polished, boiled 5 minutes	58
White, instant, boiled 1 minute	65
All bran	74

CEREAL GRAINS

Wheat Kernels	63
Bulgur	65

Couscous	66
Wheat kernels, quick cooking	75

LEGUMES

Chickpeas, dried	47
Green peas, dried	50
Peas, frozen	51
White beans, Haricot, dried	54
Chickpeas, canned	60
Pinto beans, dried	60
Garbanzo beans	61
Pinto beans, canned	64
Green peas, frozen	65
Baked beans, canned	70
Kidney beans, canned	74
Lentils, green, canned	74

PASTA

Spaghetti, brown, boiled 15 minutes	61
Spaghetti, white, boiled 15 minutes	67

SUGARS

Lactose	57

HIGH-EXTREME- GLYCAEMIC INDEX
More than 75

BREADS

Rye, whole meal	89
Barley, whole meal	93
Oat, coarse	93
Rye, crisp bread	95
Crackers, plain	100

Wheat, whole meal	100
Wheat, white bread	100
Wheat, puffed crisp bread	112
Wheat, French baguette	131

BREAKFAST CEREALS

Brown Rice	81
White Rice Polished,	81
Oat bran	85
Oats, rolled	85
Porridge oats	89
Muesli	96
Shredded Wheat (Nabisco)	97
Chinese glutenous rice	98
40% Bran Flakes	104
Weetabix	109
Rice Krispies (Kellogg's)	112
Waxy rice, boiled 14 minutes	120
Corn Flakes (Kellogg's)	121
White, instant, boiled 6 min	121
Puffed wheat	122
Puffed rice	132

CEREAL GRAINS

Wheat kernels, quick cook	75
Buckwheat	78
Sweet corn	80
Millet	103

FRUIT

Mango, ripe	81
Papaya, ripe	81
Banana, ripe	90
Raisin	93
Apricot	94

VEGETABLES

Potato, white (new), boiled	80
Carrot	92
Parsnip	97
Potato, mashed	98
Potato, russet, baked	116
Potato, peeled, sliced	117
Potato, instant	120

SUGARS

Sucrose	78
Honey	126
Glucose	138
Maltose	152

DESSERTS

Oatmeal cookies	78
Ice Cream	80
Tea cookies, 'rich'	80
Digestive biscuits	82
Shortbread	88
Tofu ice-cream substitute	155

THE PERFECT FOOD DIET – LOW-GYCAEMIC-INDEX FOOD AND EAT RIGHT FOR YOUR BLOOD TYPE

At this stage, you might feel there is some confusion between the eat-right-for-your-blood-type food menu and the low-glycaemic-index food choices you can make. Both these menu lists can be followed simultaneously without any conflict.

Our advice would be to select low-glycaemic-index food that is also listed on your beneficial list according to your particular blood type. The food target enclosed and covered below will also help you get a grip on how to select the right foods for you.

FOOD TARGET FOR LONGEVITY

We earlier covered the inverted food pyramid for longevity. Now we also provide you with another tool which is very effective in helping you to really understand which foods you must eat at every meal for optimum nutritional support. This we have called *the Food Target For Longevity*.

As with all targets the centre of the target is optimum.

- Centre – focus on fresh fruits and vegetables, preferably low glycaemic.
- Second ring – Proteins, fresh fish, beans and legumes, soy and tofu.
- Third ring out – Lean chicken, egg whites, brown rice, and incorporating low-glycaemic refined carbohydrates.
- The fourth ring out, which I think is the most effective, is white rice, milk products, red meats.
- Outside of the ring, which is to be avoided, is excessive sugar, alcohol and soft drinks, excessive dairy products, artificial sweeteners, processed packaged meats and excessive caffeine.

One of the most powerful reasons why the target works is that you can for the first time actually visualise it and incorporate it in your diet. You can instantly recognise that if you

FOOD TARGET FOR LONGEVITY & PEAK PERFORMANCE

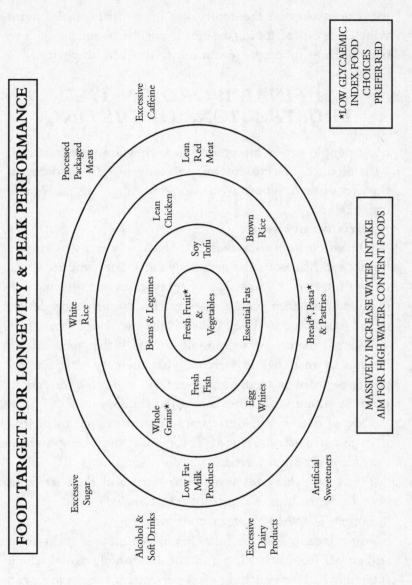

Excessive Caffeine

Processed Packaged Meats

Lean Red Meat

Lean Chicken

White Rice

Beans & Legumes

Soy Tofu

Brown Rice

Fresh Fruit★ & Vegetables

Whole Grains★

Fresh Fish

Essential Fats

Bread★, Pasta★ & Pastries

Egg Whites

Low Fat Milk Products

Artificial Sweeteners

Excessive Sugar

Alcohol & Soft Drinks

Excessive Dairy Products

★LOW GLYCAEMIC INDEX FOOD CHOICES PREFERRED

MASSIVELY INCREASE WATER INTAKE AIM FOR HIGH WATER CONTENT FOODS focus your eyes on the centre and only touch on the items which are out of focus, the result will be to finally achieve the nutrition intake for optimum health and longevity.

A FINAL WORD ON THE FRUSTRATIONS OF DIETING

Most people get to the point where they are very frustrated with dieting. They focus on yo-yoing weight or different theories of diets. There are a couple of simple things regarding diets.

Diets do not work.

The whole concept is that diets focus on scarcity, what you cannot eat. Also you subconsciously think that if you are going to go on to a diet you will have to avoid everything and feel deprived. Looking even further at this, the first three letters of the word diet are DIE, which is the ultimate in scarcity!

When a dieter says to himself or herself that they cannot eat this or that to lose weight, what their mind is actually saying to them at an unconscious level is 'I am overweight. I am fat' along with other associated things.

One of the keys to overcoming the frustration of dieting is to ask a better question. Try getting more empowered instead of dis-empowered.

Focus on what you want – to burn and shed fat from your body, to burn fat but not lose muscle.

Forget TOTALLY about your weight.

Most weight loss on other incorrect diets is short term and comes from water loss and burning muscle tissue, which is terribly bad for you and makes permanent weight loss even more difficult.

By dieting incorrectly and not nourishing your body you

are actually teaching your body to preserve its fat stores and lose muscle and water – the very things you need for permanent weight loss.

The key to successful dieting is to consume foods that will stimulate the burning of your fat stores, water to flush out the toxins and moderate exercise. Higher protein foods, lower glycaemic refined carbohydrates, lower glycaemia fresh fruits and vegetables and essential fats are all going to help burn fat. Exercise and muscle building will help accelerate burning fat stores.

It is interesting to look at the way dieters think when ordering or preparing a meal – 'will this make me fatter'?

If you continually focus on getting fatter, you are what you focus on. Educating people on how to ask a better question along the lines of 'How can I order or prepare a meal that is going to make me burn even more body fat and have increased energy, consistently through the day', is the type of question that will actually put you into a totally different frame of mind.

What better result would you get if you ask that question looking at this meal – a big, gristly saturated-fat steak and a heap of potatoes that have been fried in oil to become chips. You would automatically think 'no way', and order or prepare a meal that will increase your success in burning fat.

Part of the key to the question 'how can I burn even more fat and have increased energy' is that it pre-supposes that you are actually already burning body fat and already have lots of energy. That will give your unconscious mind the momentum that will help your conscious mind get the strength it needs to avoid such foods, no matter how good they look or smell at first.

This mind-set on your **Anti-ageing Diet** will help you

focus on the results you are going to get from a food regime that will help you to burn fat, increase your energy and extend the quality of your life.

WATER CONTENT OF FOODS

'NEXT TIME YOU'RE ON A PLANE SPILL SOME WATER ON YOUR PANTS'

Air-conditioned environments such as planes, offices and hotel rooms are dehydrating our bodies at an accelerated pace. Balanced hydration is one of the keys to assist and support the traveller and business person. Next time you're on a plane just spill some water on your pants. You will be amazed how quickly it will dry out. Your body is also drying out as quickly.

Correct hydration will make your body function more effectively, think with greater clarity, increase your energy, reduce stress, promote regular elimination and assist your muscle movement. Water makes up 70% of the planet we live on, 70% of the body we live in and should be 70% of the food we eat. A shortage of 1% or more can lead to dehydration symptoms such as headaches, fatigue, loss of appetite, heat intolerance, feeling light-headed and muscle cramps.

Ask yourself whether your food and liquid intake has water content of 70%? If the answer is no, you may find yourself to some degree dehydrated.

Most people think 'I have enough water – it is in drinks (coffee, tea, soft drinks or alcohol – all containing caffeine) I consume during the day'. Sure, they all have water in them, which is hydrating and after consumption your body's system goes above the hydrated line into optimum hydration, but at the same time the caffeine has a diuretic effect from those drinks and pulls you down slightly below the hydrated base line.

Then, if you have another drink you will go above the hydration line again, but then if the drink has caffeine in it you come down further than you did before, so your thirst continues, and it goes on and on and on. So, by the end of the day, you get to the point you are so far below the base line that not even hydrating liquids in the drinks is going to elevate you above that base line into optimum hydration.

When you spend most of your time living and working in air-conditioned environments, such as planes, offices and hotel rooms, your body loses more fluid through your skin, breathing and talking than it does through normal elimination.

If the food that you consume during the day has low water content it will compound and accelerate your body's dehydration. At the end of the day you go to sleep for 8 hours and most people don't have any liquids at all during the night. You wake up unaware you are to some degree dehydrated.

Traditionally, people start the day with breakfast of a cup of coffee and a couple of pieces of bread, which have little or no nutrients. This further contributes to your dehydration and the result is your system is dry, dry, dry.

The other popular breakfast option is a bowl of cereal with milk. If you have ever been interrupted during breakfast and come back you have to add a lot more milk to the cereal to make it palatable. With processed cereals so eager to soak up the milk just think what must be happening to your body's hydration levels when you have too much dry processed food.

To best support your body, start the day with a glass or

three of just water (preferably filtered). Then consume a very hydrating breakfast with lots of real whole fruit which has a high water content. This will assist in re-hydrating the body's biological system and moving towards optimum hydration. The soluble fibre in the fruit will also assist the body's ability to eliminate all the dry food from the previous day and prepare it for the day's intake of any dry food and for environments that are dehydrating.

If you can get the body in an exceptionally hydrated state at the start of the day, you are starting well above the hydration line and can cope much better during the course of a normal day's intake of breads, biscuits, coffee and tea without tipping the body into dehydration.

We are all aware of proper water levels as shown in other areas of our life. If you spend most of your time inside climate-controlled environments, have a look at any live plants which are there. They will be a reflection of the degree to which you are drying out. You also have to ask why imitation plants in air-conditioned environments are on the increase. It is because if they do not get constant attention with massive amounts of water real plants dry out and die.

If most people ran their cars like they ran their body, with just enough water in it so it would start and run, we would think they were crazy! We all know that if we ran our car with just enough water in it so the motor would start it would run hotter even over a short period of time. The extra heat will dramatically increase the wear and tear on the motor and the internal parts. However, we seem to have different values for the motor car than we do for the human body. If you are dehydrated ask yourself which parts are wearing out, right now. Once again, you must hydrate, really over-hydrate with appropriate food and additional water, just water.

If your body is consistently getting hydration throughout the day, it will function and perform at a higher level in all areas when in balance. With constipation and laxatives on the increase the body is just a creature of habit, so if you are eating more often and drinking more often, the body will eliminate solid waste more often when your are properly hydrated.

A tip for weight loss: next time you are feeling hungry ask yourself 'am I in need of food or are these signals telling me am I dehydrated and in need of water'?

To achieve optimum hydration an 80kg person needs to drink 8–12 (10oz glasses) of water in addition to a balanced, high-water-content food intake.

When travelling by air, an additional 400–550ml of water per hour while in the air will also assist in avoiding or minimising any jet lag. In a climate-controlled environment such as an office, hotel or home, increase your normal intake by 50%.

I imagine you may be saying to yourself, 'I will be going

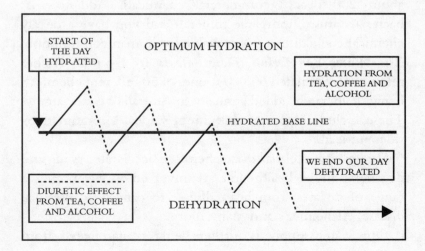

to the toilet every five minutes'. You will if you have diuretic drinks such as coffee, tea and alcohol. Proper hydration with additional water will leave your body in proper balance.

The question is, would NOW be a great time to feel even better from the benefits of optimum hydration?

NOT JUST ANY WATER

Ten years ago the prospect of drinking and paying for purified water was unheard of. Now days, it is essential to preserve good health. It is my opinion that tap water should not be drunk at all. If tap water is your only option then boil the water, expose it to the sun and aerate it before you drink it. Keep in mind that boiling it will only kill bacteria and not remove the harmful chemicals and minerals it contains.

A CHEMICAL COCKTAIL

Our drinking water today is far from being pure and contains about 200 deadly commercial chemicals. Add to that bacteria, viruses, inorganic minerals and you have a deadly chemical cocktail that is unsuitable for human consumption. **The Water You Drink, How Safe Is It?** By John Archer refers to an estimated 60,000 tonnes of 50 different chemicals being deliberately added annually to Australia's water supply. These include chlorine, aluminium sulphate, sodium fluoride and lead.

Studies indicate that these chemicals accelerate ageing and degeneration of health and are involved in promoting a range of diseases from heart disease to cancer to intestinal disease, Alzheimer's and many more.

Our water supply is further being contaminated from

other environmental mismanagement such as poor sewage treatment, farm and abattoir run off, industrial waste and toxic pollution creeping into our water.

BEWARE OF SHOWERS AND STEAM BATHS

Drinking unfiltered water is not the only way you might get these water-soluble toxins into your system. The body also absorbs water through breathing. So it is advisable to filter the water you shower in, as well as ensure if you are taking steam baths or saunas to help you detoxify that this water is properly filtered, or it may have the reverse effect.

REVERSE OSMOSIS FILTERS

Reverse osmosis is by far the most advanced technology for filtering and purifying your water. Through this process, almost all harmful bacteria, minerals and toxins are eliminated by selective separation of molecules, leaving you with clean, clear drinking water.

(see appendix for details)

Section 6

VITAMINS AND ANTIOXIDANTS ON THE ANTI-AGEING DIET

*A*ccording *to the late two-time Nobel Prize-winning scientist Linus Pauling, who lived to be 93, we could add 12 to 18 years more to our lives by taking 3200 to 12000 milligrams of Vitamin C a day.*

A study recently published in the Lancet reported that elderly people taking multivitamins with minerals had improved immune function and had 50% fewer sick days.

Dr Eric Rimm, in a Harvard study on the role of Vitamin E in heart disease, found that 'the risk in not taking vitamin E was equivalent to the risk of smoking'.

More than 100 studies have shown that people with high levels of beta-carotene in their diet and blood are only half as likely to develop cancer in the lungs, mouth, throat, oesophagus, larynx, stomach, breast, or bladder.

According to a 20-year study at the University of Mississippi, low levels of Vitamin C and E are to blame for many cardiovascular problems.

About 120 separate studies say that Vitamin C is a virtual 'vaccination' against cancer, according to Berkley epidemiologist Dr Gladys Black.

Due to all the recent publicity and push by vitamin companies, one of the most widely understood yet still confusing components of **The Anti-ageing Diet** is vitamins and anti-oxidants. We have already covered in an earlier chapter the Free-Radical Theory of Ageing, and vitamins and anti-oxidants are the most powerful combatants of this cause of ageing.

There are many different vitamins and antioxidants (not all vitamin are antioxidants). The most important antioxidant vitamins are Vitamin C, Vitamin E and Vitamin A or Beta-carotene.

They are called antioxidants because of their unique ability to deactivate harmful free radicals that accumulate in our bodies, in addition to their ability to maintain the structure and function of our cells.

In essence, oxygen creates these free radicals, be it through our immune system battling foreign substances, or even through strenuous exercise. It is these antioxidant vitamins that halt the destructive path of free radicals and stabilise them back to normal, healthy molecules.

THE GREAT LIE: YOU CAN GET ALL THE NUTRITION YOU NEED FROM FOOD

Now, it's certainly possible to get enough C, E and A in your daily diet – if you are measuring 'enough' by the US Department of Agriculture daily recommended allowance (RDA). Calculated by government officials, RDA standards are just enough to avoid common vitamin-deficient diseases, such as scurvy, rickets or beriberi. They do not account for what is needed to maintain maximum health.

RDA are far too low for optimal health.

What you should be striving for is optimal daily allowances

(ODA) in your **Anti-ageing Diet**, which requires between 5 and 100 times RDA requirements. According to Linus Pauling, the amounts being recommended to the public are hardly enough to reap any Anti-ageing benefits at all.

And despite the RDA standards being so low, a disturbing reality is that many people do not get enough vitamins to meet even these skimpy requirements.

If, however, 'ordinary poor health' is not good enough for you and you wish to live **The Anti-ageing Diet** from now on, then you should begin to find out what your current base line deficiencies are today and seek the advice of a qualified Anti-ageing specialist.

The right quantities of supplemental doses of E, C, beta-carotene and CoQ-10 could literally save your life – while helping to make your life worth living.

VITAMIN C: IT'S SO POWERFUL

It has been known by scientists for years that megadoses of Vitamin C offer innumerable benefits, from overcoming the common cold to stopping the onslaught of cancer. But it is only recently that the full range of this vitamin's benefits have become accepted by the wider community.

Vitamin C is now credited with the following:

- Fights the ageing effects of air pollution, radiation and chemotherapy
- Is anti-inflammatory, reducing the degenerative symptoms typical of arthritis
- Stimulates collagen production to keep skin youthful and flexible
- Helps protect arteries from hardening

- Increases HDL cholesterol, protecting from heart diseases
- Helps the body absorb iron needed for energy and brain function
- Helps synthesise carnitine – fat-burning nutrient
- Helps overcome allergies as an antihistamine
- Activates folic acid to protect the lining of the stomach and prevent the formation of polyps and other pre-cancerous conditions
- Prevents cancer by boosting the immune systems and white blood cells
- Stimulates the adrenal glands, improving mental alertness and protecting from stress.

One of the most interesting facts about Vitamin C is that most mammals produce their own. Only humans and a few other creatures have lost this capacity in the evolutionary process. A 65 kg mammal manufactures about 10,000mg of vitamin C a day – that's equivalent to the amount of Vitamin C you'll find in 100 glasses of orange juice!

Under stress, both human and animal bodies need extra Vitamin C to counter the age-accelerating effects of free radicals that stress creates.

As a result, and according to Dr Emanual Cheraskin, a professor at the University of Alabama, 'virtually nobody gets enough Vitamin C'.

According to UCLA researcher Dr James Enstrom, you can expect even greater health benefits from taking Vitamin C supplements than you can from lowering cholesterol and cutting fat in your diet. He believes that people who take Vitamin C can expect to live longer, even if they smoke, eat high-fat diets, are overweight and fail to exercise!

With all this overwhelming evidence, Vitamin C is an essential component of your daily **Anti-Ageing Diet**.

VITAMIN C AND HEART DISEASE

Dr Matthias Rath, author of *Eradicating Heart Disease*, believes the lack of certain nutrients is the essential cause of most cardiovascular diseases – particularly the thinning of the arterial walls. Vitamin C acts as a stabilising nutrient, guaranteeing biochemical balance. Blood walls become very fragile when there is a Vitamin C deficiency.

Reinforced blood vessels is the basic protection against arteriosclerotic deposits and cardiovascular disease. With low Vitamin C in the diet for many years, the repair function goes on and on, resulting in large quantities of fatty lipoproteins being deposited on the blood vessel walls, eventually closing them off completely. Cardiovascular failure is then right around the corner.

VITAMIN C AND DIABETES

Diabetics, in particular, could benefit from large doses of Vitamin C. Their bodies have greater difficulty absorbing Vitamin C in the cell.

In their case, insulin and glucose compete for the job of carrying Vitamin C to the cell, a competition that may result in the exact opposite occurring – insufficient Vitamin C being carried by either substance.

This results in diabetics often having reduced levels of Vitamin C even when their intake is far above the recommended level.

Therefore, it is particularly important for diabetics who

are following the **Anti-ageing Diet** to increase their intake, directed by a specialist.

VITAMIN C AND CANCER

Vitamin C not only prevents the activation of free radicals, but researchers believe it is essential to prevent the formation of cancer-causing particles called nitrosamines. It helps stop nitrates and other substances from becoming carcinogenic, and acts as the first line of defence against the 'ageing-disease' cancer.

The late Scottish cancer specialist Ewan Cameron was one of the first physicians to notice low levels of Vitamin C in his cancer patients.

After treating his patients with high levels of Vitamin C – around 10,000 milligrams per day – he became convinced of its anti-cancer properties.

For example, one patient had lymphatic cancer and was admitted to hospital for radiation therapy. A two-week backlog for this treatment resulted in his prescribing an intra-venous alternative of 10g of Vitamin C per day. By the time radiation therapy was available, it was no longer necessary: the signs of his cancer had vanished and x-rays had shown a significant improvement.

Vitamin C is not a sure-fire cure for cancer, but numerous reports and studies show it has an obvious positive effect on this debilitating disease.

VITAMIN C AND ANTI-AGEING

Vitamin C virtually reverses the biological clock by rejuve-nating white blood cells. One of the most remarkable studies concerning Vitamin C was conducted at UCLA in 1992. The diets of 11,000 people were studied over a 10-year period. The results? Overall Vitamin C consumption increased life expectancy of women by 1 year and men by 6.

HOW MUCH C ON YOUR ANTI-AGEING DIET?

Vitamin C is water-soluble. It leaves the body easily through urination. This is both good and bad. It means you cannot overdose on it, but on the other hand, you must take it frequently to keep your body's Vitamin C level high.

The **Anti-ageing Diet** recommendation would be 1000-2000mg per day depending on your body mass, and even higher doses if you're feeling sick or under stress. Many people have found at the first warning signs of colds or flu, or other illness, that taking 5000mg to start with and 1000-2000mg every hour after will 'blast' the illness out of their bodies.

This may cause mild diarrhoea or nausea and heartburn. Everyone's bowel tolerance is different, but up to 2000mg per day causes no reaction.

Smoking, drinking, breathing polluted air or long periods of stress are not recommended as part of your **Anti-ageing Diet**, however, if you find yourself in this situation, or you are using birth control pills you must obtain extra amounts of Vitamin C. This also applies for women during menstruation.

Headaches are sometimes a result of stressful conditions. Vitamin C may be a better alternative than a headache tablet.

It is also a good idea to drink a large glass of water or juice each time you take high doses of Vitamin C.

VITAMIN E

While Vitamin C is water-soluble (found in the water parts of our cells), Vitamin E is fat-soluble. Vitamin E inhibits fats cells from becoming 'infected' with oxygen and turning rancid. In a sense, Vitamin E is our first line of defence against free-radical damage to fats in the cell walls.

Numerous studies have shown Vitamin E to:

- Prevent heart attack and stroke
- Clear arteries of plaque
- Increase immunity
- Inhibit the growth of cancer cells
- Prevent the progress of brain disease
- Ease arthritis
- Increase circulation to the leg arteries
- Improve blood circulation
- Boost healing of scars and burns

VITAMIN E AND HEART DISEASE

You may already be aware there are two types of cholesterol – HDL (good) and LDL (bad) cholesterol. Vitamin E protects against the oxidisation of the LDL cholesterol. We now believe that LDL cholesterol poses no particular danger to our bodies until it oxidises or turns rancid. Once it has turned rancid it becomes able to infiltrate the artery walls, where it builds up as plaque and blocks blood flow.

According to Dr Ishawal Jailal, of the University of Texas Southwestern Medical Centre, subjects who took 800IU of Vitamin E daily for 3 months cut the rate of LDL oxidisation by 40%. It is also his opinion that you will begin to see benefits in this regard with daily E supplements as low as 400IU.

Similarly, a Harvard study of Vitamin E showed that the risk of heart disease with people taking between 100 and 250IU was 41% lower that those who did not take Vitamin E.

E-takers also had a 29% lower risk of stroke.

VITAMIN E AND DIABETES

Diabetics will experience particular benefit from Vitamin E. It inhibits the oxidative reaction that leads to protein linking in the blood stream to excess sugar.

VITAMIN E AND CANCER

Many studies have shown the strong link between Vitamin E and battling cancer. A national Cancer Institute study revealed that when people took an extra 100IU of Vitamin E their risk of cancer was reduced by 50%. Dr Blumberg, at Tufts University, says Vitamin E helps prevent cancer in 3 steps.

- Prevents the formation of carcinogens
- Enhances the body's immune system
- Shields the cells from free radicals

HOW VITAMIN E FIGHTS AGEING

Vitamin E returns an ageing person's immunity to youthful levels.

Dr Simin Meydani, at Tufts University, administered between 400 and 800IU of Vitamin E daily to people over 60. Although their immune response had been declining,

Vitamin E reversed that tr[...]
responses back to youthful [...]
people who were considered [...]
standards.

In our modern world, wl[...]
environmental hazards attac[...]
protection of Vitamin E. Vita[...]
isation of the fat molecules [...]
damage they cause.

with meals. Up to 80[...]
tends to have mil[...]
so is not recor[...]
Megados[...]
may be [...]
press[...]

E AND E[...]

Vitamin E is especially important for those who exercise frequently. Ironically, while exercise helps to prevent ageing, it also increases the risk of ageing. When we exercise, we create more free radicals, so the more aerobic activity you do the higher doses of Vitamin E you should include in your daily diet.

HOW MUCH E ON YOUR ANTI-AGEING DIET?

Vitamin E has virtually no side-effects at optimal doses. Although you get some E in foods, to experience its Anti-ageing effects you must take supplements. To get the 400IU that most Anti-ageing specialists recommend and which we recommend as part of your **Anti-ageing Diet**, you would need to consume two quarts of corn oil, more than five pounds of wheat germ, eight cups of almonds, or 22 cups of peanuts. If you chose the latter route, you would also be consuming 22,250 calories and 1912 grams of fat – hardly a healthy choice!

The best way to take E is in two 200IU doses each day

...0IU is a safe dose, but more than 400IU
...d anti-clotting effects like those of aspirin,
...mmended for people facing surgery.
...es of Vitamin E of 2000IU to 3200IU, however,
...toxic, causing headaches, diarrhoea and high blood
...ure. These levels should be avoided.

Once you start taking Vitamin E, expect to continue for a lifetime, because it can take up to two years before the heart-helping benefits of this vitamin reach their optimal level.

BETA-CAROTENE AND VITAMIN A: THE SUPREME ANTIOXIDANT

Beta-carotene has become one of the most powerful anti-oxidants on the market today. It is able to convert itself into Vitamin A in the body without risking any of Vitamin A's toxic side-effects at levels higher than 5000IU.

Beta-carotene has many Anti-ageing benefits such as:

- Preventing lung, stomach and breast cancer
- Preventing stroke and heart attack
- Stopping the build-up of cholesterol
- Destroying tumour cell
- Strengthening the immune system
- Preventing cataracts and improving night vision.

BETA-CAROTENE AND CANCER

Studies at the Johns Hopkins Schools of Hygiene and Public Health found that people with low levels of beta-carotene were 4 times as likely to develop a common form of smoking-related lung cancer as those with higher beta-carotene levels.

Beta-carotene also help to block cervical cancer. A six-year Australian study found that women who already had breast cancer had a survival rate 12 times higher if they consumed high levels of beta-carotene.

BETA-CAROTENE AND HEART ATTACK

A Harvard University study by Dr Charles Hennekens found that men who took 50mg of beta-carotene every second day for 6 years had only half as many fatal heart attacks, strokes and other heart-disease incidents as men who took a placebo during that same period.

BETA-CAROTENE AND ANTI-AGEING

Like vitamins C and E, beta-carotene helps fight free radicals. It is also used by our bodies to manufacture Vitamin A, which prevents ageing by boosting our immune system. Vitamin A helps keep skin smooth and young looking, as well as strengthens our bones.

HOW TO TAKE BETA-CAROTENE ON THE ANTI-AGEING DIET

It's easier to get beta-carotene in your diet than Vitamin C or E from dark yellow, orange or dark green vegetables or fruit. The human body can, however, more easily absorb beta-carotene in supplements than in natural food. Heavy cooking destroys beta-carotene. Foods such as sweet potatoes, carrots, greens and spinach lose beta-carotene value when cooked.

Take 10-15mg a day of beta-carotene supplements divided in doses with meals, because you need fats to digest it. Beta-carotene appears to be non-toxic. Even though high concentrations of Vitamin A can have adverse effects, the body never manufactures its own toxic quantities of A no matter how much beta-carotene you take. The only side-effect may be a slight yellowing of the skin, which only happens at extremely high doses.

COENZYME Q-10: THE MIRACLE HEART MEDICINE

Although many people have never heard of Coenzyme Q-10, millions of people in Japan and Europe take it for congestive heart failure and a variety of other illnesses.

Coenzyme Q-10 is a highly fat-soluble molecule usually found in the mitochondria where it manufactures ATP (adenosine triphosphate). ATP is the basic energy molecule for the entire human body. Coenzyme Q-10's health benefits lie in its ability to help produce energy. It is therefore most important and needed in greater quantities in muscles and tissues that are most active all the time, such as the heart, liver and immune system.

Like many biochemicals, Coenzyme Q-10 declines rapidly, beginning at age 20 and dropping almost 80% by around 50.

Supplementation is not the only way to increase Coenzyme Q-10, and many studies point to increased rigorous exercise as a way to increase our own levels of this enzyme.

COENZYME Q-10 AND THE ANTI-AGEING DIET

It's advisable to take Coenzyme Q-10 supplements if you're 50 or older, especially if you are prone to heart problems. Healthy, younger people should begin with 30mg daily but people with a specific problem might want to increase this from 50-150 mg per day, depending on your Anti-ageing specialist's advice.

Unless you have a severe Coenzyme Q-10 deficiency you probably won't notice its effects right away. It may take 1-3 months for the enzyme to begin to effect your heart, and its impact on energy or immune system may even be more subtle.

Your body manufactures its own Coenzyme Q-10. For this process, it requires B group vitamins: B6, B12, niacin and folic acid. You can also find Coenzyme Q-10 in many types of food, such as fatty fish (mackerel, sardines), organ meats such as heart, liver and kidney, soy oil and peanuts. Again, you'd need to eat half a kilogram of sardines or a kilogram of peanuts just to get 30mg of Coenzyme Q-10, so supplements are probably your best bet. Just be sure you're taking an oil-based capsule or adding a little fat (ie olive oil) to the dry tablets.

OTHER IMPORTANT VITAMINS FOR YOUR ANTI-AGEING DIET

VITAMIN D

The best way to get adequate amounts of Vitamin D is from sunlight, allowing the skin to manufacture its own quantities. It can also be obtained through food or supplements.

Suggested Anti-ageing Diet doses 400-500IU.

VITAMIN K

Amongst other qualities, Vitamin K helps detoxify the liver, ease bruising and prevent gallstones, jaundice and ulcers.

Suggested Anti-ageing doses 40–70mcg per day

VITAMINS:

B1–Thiamine The body can only store small amounts of B1 and must be supplemented daily. During stress and depression the body rapidly uses B1, so extra amounts must be taken. This includes periods of strenuous exercise, pregnancy, or alcohol consumption.

Suggested Anti-ageing doses 1000mcg per day.

B2–Riboflavin

This is essential for good eye sight, young-looking skin and cellular regeneration. Daily supplements are needed for increased stamina and vitality. A B2 deficiency can also result in baldness, falling hair, oily skin, acne, ulcers, arthritic conditions, Parkinson's disease, influenza, diabetes and physical exhaustion. Women on oestrogen supplements need to take B2.

Suggested Anti-ageing doses 100–300mg per day.

B3–Niacin

Niacin is involved in the energy-producing functions of the cells. A niacin deficiency may show up as general fatigue, indigestion or poor appetite. Too much sugar or high-glycaemic-index carbohydrate foods will lead to a deficiency, and so will strenuous exercise.

Suggested Anti-ageing doses 200mg per day.

B5–Pantothenic acid

B5 is essential for proper digestion and breakdown of fats and controls the use of cholesterol. It improves the condition of hair, eyes and nerves. A deficiency may lead to ulcers and reduced antibodies to fight infection.

B5 prevents the onset of premature ageing, wrinkly skin, baldness, arthritis and retarded growth. It also protects the body from cellular damage from radiation.

Suggested Anti–ageing doses 2400mg per day.

VITAMIN B6

B6 is essential for production of antibodies and conversion of protein to amino acids. A B6 deficiency may lead to irritability, adrenal exhaustion, headaches, poor concentration and memory, and poorly functioning pituitary gland.

Suggested Anti–ageing doses 50mg daily.

VITAMIN B12

B12, amongst other things, is required for the proper synthesis of Vitamin C and iron. All animals except humans can synthesise their own B12.

Suggested Anti–ageing doses 100mcg.

VITAMIN H-BIOTIN

Biotin assists the body to produce a natural supply of lecithin, which is used by the body to control the level of fat and cholesterol in the blood. Antibiotics deplete the body of biotin. Biotin and all other B vitamins work in harmony. Additional biotin may be required during pregnancy.

Suggested Anti–ageing doses 300mcg.

CHOLINE

Assists in rejuvenating aged kidneys, liver, the muscles of the brain and heart. It is also important in the storage of calcium, which is important for the prevention of osteoporosis.

Suggested Anti–ageing doses 1000mg per day.

INOSITOL

Inositol is important for the proper functioning of the nervous system. Pesticides use an ingredient which paralyses the vital amount of inositol in insects, which kills them. Similar effects are caused to the human body's supply of inositol from exposure to pesticides in our food and environment.

Suggested Anti-ageing doses 50mg per day.

P.A.B.A.

This is essential for preventing such ageing problems as fading hair colour and skin pigment disorders. It is often used in sunscreens.

Suggested Anti-ageing doses 50 mg per day.

MORE DANGEROUS THAN CHOLESTEROL

It is now recognised that elevated levels of homocystene level in the blood are a major risk factor for heart disease. Some doctors are even stating that high homocystene levels are a greater risk to heart disease than high cholesterol.

Homocystene is produced in the body as a by-product of metabolism.

FOLIC ACID

When homocystene builds up, it can effectively be metabolised with additional quantities of folic acid, B6 and B12. Involving more than 80,000 nurses, researchers at Harvard School of Public Health found a 45% reduced risk of coronary heart disease with intakes of both folic acid and B6.

Suggested Anti-ageing doses 800mcg per day.

A WORD OF WARNING

The suggested Anti-ageing doses outlined in this diet are based on doses provided to the average healthy adult.

Incorrect uses and dosage for you may be harmful, and no vitamin regime should be undertaken without first consulting your Anti-ageing specialist to ensure no other medical condition exists that may be compromised by taking vitamins.

NATURAL VS SYNTHETIC VITAMINS AND MINERALS

Natural vitamins are derived from our food. Synthetic vitamins are those manufactured in a laboratory. Is there really a difference between these two?

Due to the over-processing of our foods, our diets are often vitamin and mineral deficient, and in most cases we have no option but to supplement by using synthetic vitamins and minerals. Critics claim synthetic vitamins cannot be absorbed by the body and may themselves be a waste of money or toxic to the body.

A basic guideline to follow when shopping for your vitamins is that not all vitamins are the same and that cheaper is not better. Cheap vitamins lack bioavailability and cannot be metabolised or absorbed.

To check the quality of your vitamins you should be able to break it in your fingers or with a dull knife, or it should easily dissolve in a glass of warm water. Also check your urine – if it is bright yellow it means your body is absorbing the vitamin's nutrients.

MINERALS ON THE ANTI-AGEING DIET

E very living cell on this planet depends on minerals for proper function and structure. Minerals are needed for the proper composition of body fluids, the formation of blood and bone, the maintenance of healthy nerve function and the regulation of muscle tone, including that of the muscles of the cardiovascular system. Like vitamins, minerals function as coenzymes, enabling the body to perform its functions, including energy production, growth and healing.

WHY DO WE NEED MINERALS?

The human body, as all of nature, must maintain its proper chemical balance. This balance depends on the levels of different minerals in the body and especially the ratios of certain mineral levels to one another. The level of each mineral in the body has an effect on every other, so if one is out of balance, all mineral levels are affected. If not corrected, this can start a chain reaction of imbalances that lead to illness.

WHAT ARE MINERALS?

Minerals are naturally occurring elements found in the earth. Rock formations are made up of mineral salts. Over millions of years the rock formations are eroded into dust and sand, forming the basis of soil. The mineral salts in the soil are then passed from the soil to plants. The plants are eaten by herbivorous animals. We obtain these minerals by consuming plants or herbivorous animals.

There are two groups of minerals – macrominerals and microminerals.

Macrominerals include calcium, magnesium, sodium, potassium and phosphorous. Microminerals include boron, chromium, copper, iodine, iron, manganese, molybdenum, selenium, sulphur, vanadium and zinc.

One of the biggest mistakes you may ever make is to believe in the myth of 'a balanced diet'. Even if you were to follow a diet of carefully selected supermarket foods and inorganic fruit and vegetables, supplemented with bottled vitamins and minerals, you will still be grossly deficient in many vital minerals and trace elements.

The basis for all life on earth is the soil. A lack of any nutrient or trace mineral in the soil directly translates into an inadequacy in the vegetation supported by the soil and in the animals supported by that vegetation.

Primitive people who hunted and gathered uncultivated, natural foods, very rarely became ill or contracted diseases. The soil was mineral rich. In nature, minerals are constantly added to the soil by the breakdown of bedrock, as vegetative processes and erosion take place. Enzymes, earthworms, and micro-organisms break inorganic minerals down into forms easily assimilated by plants.

In a balanced ecosystem, plant life is strong and possesses the vitality to be naturally resistant to insects and disease. Disease and infestation only occurs as a natural adjustment to an unbalanced ecosystem. The same law applies to animals and humans.

7 MAGIC ANTI-AGEING MINERALS – THE TRUE FOUNTAIN OF YOUTH!

In the sacred valley of Vilcabamba, Ecuador, the mountain people often live well beyond 100 years, remaining strong, healthy, sexual and actively working until the last months of life.

One of their secrets to such a long and productive life is the 7 magic minerals found in their food and water. Unlike the body mineral content of western industrialised people, the Vilcabambans show perfect ratios of these essential minerals in their hair-mineral analysis. They are not subject to degenerative diseases such as cancer, diabetes, heart disease and arteriosclerosis ... the minerals they drink in their water supply seem to be their natural protection.

Their water has the perfect balance of the 7 magic minerals of longevity – selenium, chromium, zinc, manganese, potassium, calcium and magnesium.

HERE'S THE BAD NEWS ...

Our bodies cannot produce their own minerals, and it is almost impossible to obtain the amount of minerals needed for optimum health through diet alone.

Since our body cannot produce its own minerals, minerals must be constantly supplied to it, primarily from colloidal mineral-rich plants such as fruit and vegetables. The problem is, however, that the food we eat, even if it includes a lot of grains, fruits and vegetables, is significantly lacking in good mineral content because the soil from which it is grown is significantly depleted of minerals, especially the trace elements.

Most fruits, vegetables and meats today may look good, but they lack flavour. This is because they contain only a fraction of the necessary minerals. Minerals are what give foods their natural flavour.

Today we would have to eat at least 10 apples to get the same nutritional value that was in one apple 100 years ago.

Looking at the difference between organic and inorganic grown vegetables we get the idea of just how depleted our soils are in the various minerals.

For example:

% of dry weight		Mileq./100g dry wgt		Parts per million of dry matter			
	Calcium	Magnesium	Boron	Manganese	Iron	Copper	Cobalt
Lettuce							
Organic	71.00	49.30	37.00	169.00	516.00	60.00	0.19
Inorganic	16.00	13.10	6.00	1.00	9.00	3.00	0.00
Tomatoes							
Organic	23.00	59.20	36.00	68.00	1938.00	53.00	0.63
Inorganic	4.50	4.50	5.00	1.00	1.00	0.00	0.00
Spinach							
Organic	96.00	203.90	88.00	117.00	1584.00	32.00	0.25
Inorganic	47.50	64.60	12.00	1.00	19.00	0.50	0.20

This is listing just a few of the minerals on just three staple vegetables in our daily diets. By far the most amazing is spinach. One would have to eat a huge quantity of inorganic spinach to get an adequate dose of iron.

A summary of the United States Senate document #264 of the '74 Congress, 2nd Session, states that laboratory tests prove that US farm and range soils are depleted of minerals and the grains, fruits and vegetables, nuts, eggs and even milk are not what they were a few generations ago. It also states that people who eat these foods develop mineral deficiency diseases which can only be corrected by including mineral supplements in their diet. It says that 99% of the population were deficient in minerals at the time of the report. And that was 39 years ago!

SICK SOIL MEANS SICK ANIMALS AND SICK PEOPLE

Here is something so incredible, you probably won't believe it ... What has killed more Americans in the past 57 years than wars, Hitler's Holocaust, and the Hiroshima atomic bombings combined? The gross deficiency of one single mineral in our diets! Magnesium!

Mineral deficiency is a growing epidemic. Years ago you heard about people in various localities with mineral deficiencies and illness, due to poor soil, perhaps iodine or selenium. Now that people get their foods from varied sources, we all share deficiencies, so these connections aren't noticed today.

One person every 10 minutes dies of heart disease in Australia today. Cancer is increasing. One person in three will get cancer! Almost everyone you know has some chronic health problem and complains about headaches, digestive trouble, backache, allergies, lack of energy etc.

People are now consuming pills, drugs, vitamins and herbal remedies at record rates.

So why does the situation continue to get worse each year? Many experts now conclude that our increasingly deficient food supplies are the true cause of much of our suffering. And vitamins are ineffective in improving our health without minerals.

All nutrients such as vitamins, proteins, enzymes, amino acids, carbohydrates, and fatty acids need minerals before they can be properly utilised by the body. Although vitamins have received much more attention than minerals, many people are surprised to learn that most vitamins can be manufactured within our body, while minerals can only be obtained from outside the body, primarily from plant-based foods.

YOUR DOG IS HEALTHIER THAN YOU ARE . . .

Fifty years ago, a law was passed by the US Congress requiring dog food to be updated every three years to the latest nutritional standards.

So now dog food is loaded with minerals and is greatly superior to the average American diet. Have you noticed that the only dogs that actually get sick are those that are fed table scraps?

Many veterinarians advise that you should never feed your pet human food if you want it to be healthy. If someone tells you their dog has arthritis or some other 'human disease', ask them what they feed it. Many animal and livestock disorders were easily eliminated years ago, just by adding a few inexpensive minerals to the animals' feed.

DO YOU HAVE A MINERAL DEFICIENCY?

Below is a simple test to determine if you are mineral deficient. If you underline 3 or more in one of the groups, you may have the indicated deficiency. This is meant as a guide ONLY. You should seek Anti-ageing medical advice before you begin self-diagnosing your symptoms. See a doctor if you are in doubt.

GROUP 1:

Aching joints, kidney stones, heel of bone spurs, twitches or facial tics, receding gums, gingivitis, pyorrhoea, insomnia, spinal curvature, PMS, osteoporosis, Paget's disease, bursitis, painful tendons, leg or menstrual cramps, dental cavities, hypertension, irritability, arthritic conditions, gnarled knuckles etc.

Deficiency: CALCIUM

GROUP 2:

Irregular heart beats, cold extremities, or just cold a lot, constipation, heart disease, hyperactivity, osteoporosis, clogged arteries, high blood pressure, fatigue.

Deficiency: MAGNESIUM

MAGNESIUM

Magnesium deficiency reads like the who's who of old age. Approximately two-thirds of people who need magnesium the most consume less than 75% of the RDA. Diabetics, people on low-calorie diets, alcoholics, strenuous exercisers and those taking prescribed heart medication need to be aware of their need for greater magnesium intakes.

Not only does it protect against heart disease, it also fights chronic fatigue syndrome, lowers blood pressure and prevents re-occurring kidney stones. Most importantly, however, it plays a central role in keeping bones strong and with calcium helps prevent osteoporosis.

Most people are aware of the need to increase their intake of calcium, particularly with age, however, few people realise the importance of using magnesium with calcium (and Vitamin D) to keep bones strong.

Without magnesium, taking calcium
heart attack and stroke.

Magnesium also works with calcium to ease t
of PMS. Refined sugar and dairy products – wh
women crave during this time – actually interferes w
absorption of magnesium, creating a deficiency that
exacerbate PMS symptoms. The anxiety, irritability and
mood swing common to this time can be attributed to insufficient magnesium available to produce adequate levels of
dopamine – a neurotransmitter that acts like a natural tran-
quilliser and mood elevator.

Another benefit of magnesium is the relief it offers to
sufferers of chronic fatigue syndrome (CFS). In a study of
32 people, 15 were given magnesium and the other 17 a
placebo. Of the 15, 12 people reported feeling better, of the
17 only 3 felt better.

MAGNESIUM ON YOUR
ANTI-AGEING DIET

If you don't eat magnesium-rich foods, you should be taking
200–300mg supplement each day. A typical multivitamin
generally only includes 100mg so you may need an additional supplement.

Magnesium oxide is the only form of magnesium to
avoid, because most people just don't tolerate it well.

Most people can tolerate up to 500mg if they have normal
kidney function. People with kidney or heart conditions
should consult an Anti-ageing specialist before considering
magnesium supplements.

Ideally, you should take half as much magnesium as
calcium, but many people seem to take only one quarter as

0mg of calcium you will need
ps more if your diet is high in
ld not be if you are following

tiredness, recurrent yeast infec-
ry of cystic fibrosis, muscular
oblems, cataracts, liver problems
ss (imbalance), low resistance to

Deficiency: SELENIUM

SELENIUM

Selenium is known as the anti-virus supplement, as it keeps
our immune systems functioning at youthful levels.

Will Taylor, of the University of Georgia College of
Pharmacy, suggests that selenium may be a powerful
weapon in the fight against AIDS. The HIV virus depletes
selenium supply in the cell, and when this occurs the virus
replicates itself and breaks out of the cell to search for more
selenium.

Dr Gerhard Schrauzerat, of the University of California,
San Deigo, has reported a similar phenomenon. 'As long as
there is enough selenium around in the cells the virus
behaves itself.'

Declining immunity is one of the trademarks of ageing,
leaving people vulnerable to cancer, heart disease and other
illnesses. A University of Brussels researcher found that
giving older patients 100mcg of selenium daily for six
months increased the body's lymphocyte invaders by some

79%, reaching levels typically associated with the young.

After the age of 60, our selenium levels drop by 7% and after 75 they drop around 24%.

A Dutch study of 3000 older people found that those with higher level of selenium had only half as great a chance of getting cancer as their low-selenium counterparts.

Selenium also prevents blood cells from sticking together, reducing the risk of blood clot, heart attack and stroke. It is also a powerful antioxidant that helps detoxify your body. Along with glutathione, selenium helps remove toxic heavy metals such as mercury, lead and cadmium, carrying them to the urine where they are flushed out of the system.

SELENIUM ON YOUR ANTI-AGEING DIET

You can get natural selenium in grains, sunflower seeds, garlic and seafood, particularly swordfish, and oysters. The best natural source of selenium, however, is brazil nuts in the shell. Each unshelled nut contains about 100mcg of selenium.

If you're not going to eat brazil nuts every day then you need to supplement between 100–200mcg a day. High doses of selenium can be toxic, where cases of 1000mcg per day have resulted in complications. Yet Japanese fishermen consume high quantities of selenium – around 500mcg – without apparent harm. Again, check with your Anti-ageing specialist if in doubt.

GROUP 4:
Chronic tiredness, dizziness upon standing or getting up,

frequent urination, always/never thirsty, impotence, infertility, menstrual distress, liver problems, digestive difficulty, alcoholism, Alzheimer's, hypoglycaemia, diabetes, kidney failure.

Deficiency: CHROMIIUM and/or VANADIUM

CHROMIIUM

People, especially those over 35, become less efficient at using insulin to transport sugar. As a result your blood will experience higher levels of blood sugar and insulin – both substances extremely bad for your heart, arteries and metabolism.

This condition starts a vicious cycle – the more sugar your blood contains the more insulin your pancreas releases, and the more insulin you have the more resistant your cells become to it, making matters worse for transporting sugar.

Researchers believe that 4 out of 5 people could benefit by including chromium in their diets. Another important role of chromium is in synthesising protein and in the transport of this protein into muscle cells, aiding the development of muscle tissue.

In a recent study, eight people with glucose intolerance were administered 200mcg of chromium a day for five weeks. Of those eight, seven showed dramatic improvements in blood sugar levels.

A lowering of insulin levels in your blood helps prevent insulin from attacking your artery walls and prevents the onset of arteriosclerosis. Chromium also works to lower LDL cholesterol while raising HDL cholesterol. For 3 decades, researchers have known that people who died of heart disease had abnormally low levels of chromium.

At Auburn University, Alabama, men tested with chromium supplements experienced a 14% drop in their total cholesterol.

CHROMIUM ON YOUR ANTI-AGEING DIET

When taking chromium supplements, look for an organic, rather than inorganic, supplement. Your body will do far better absorbing the organic chromium and make more use of it.

Anti-ageing scientists generally recommend about 200mcg for both adults and teenagers. Diabetics, however, should not alter their intake of chromium without consulting their specialist as it might affect their need for insulin.

Chromium should begin to lower blood sugar within a few days or weeks and within a few weeks to months you should begin to see lower cholesterol and triglycerides.

It is unlikely that you will ever overdose on chromium. Conceivably you could take 300 times the recommended dose without ill effect, however, this is certainly not recommended.

It is ironic that many symptoms of chromium deficiency – insulin resistance, mature/adult-onset diabetes, rising cholesterol and triglycerides – are often mistaken for the symptoms of normal ageing, where these can be avoided.

GROUP 5:
Premature greying of hair, anaemia, wrinkles, sagging skin, thin skin, family history of aneurism, liver cirrhosis, arthritic conditions.
Deficiency: COPPER

COPPER ON YOUR ANTI-AGEING DIET

Around 2mg per day.

SO WHAT IS THE ANSWER?

For centuries our parents have been telling us, 'eat your vegetables'. Well, the advice today is, 'TAKE YOUR MINERALS'!

The US Government said it: 99% of us aren't getting enough. They also said that a mineral deficiency is worse than a vitamin deficiency. If you think you are getting your minerals from a balanced diet ... think again.

Mineral supplements will give your body the minerals that it requires. However, supplemental minerals should always be taken in balanced amounts or they may be ineffective or even harmful. It is not enough to simply start taking supplements. Some forms of mineral supplements are harder for your body to digest and absorb. And like most biochemical substances, minerals don't act alone. They interact and engage in a complicated series of transactions with other minerals, vitamins and hormones.

YOUR BODY IS LIKE A FINELY TUNED ORCHESTRA

For a symphony orchestra to produce beautiful music, all instruments need to be finely tuned and be played perfectly in tune and in time. This is exactly the way the human body works. There is very little point in partly supplementing or partly being on **The Anti-ageing Diet**, because this will not produce the best result or the result you may wish for.

You need a good understanding of how each supplement works and how it interacts with other nutrients you consume and the effect all of this has on the functioning and production of hormones.

The Anti-ageing Diet recommends that your daily mineral supplementation be administered by a qualified practitioner.

Depending on your age, gender, stage of life and lifestyle, you may have different needs for varying levels of minerals. The best way to identify any deficiencies is to test your blood or urine for mineral levels. An analysis will provide a record that reflects normal and abnormal metabolism, assimilation and exposure.

A proper biochemical assessment of your blood sample is displayed on a large TV monitor which shows the undernourished cells leading to malnutrition and disease. Further tests after a reasonable period on your **Anti-ageing Diet** including mineral supplements will show a return to more healthy blood, reflecting a healthy biological terrain and healthy cells.

Section 8

HORMONES ON THE ANTI-AGEING DIET

GROW YOUNG WITH HGH

A 60-year-old man becomes Mr Physical Fitness.
A 50-year-old college teacher regains the face and figure of her modelling days.
A 43-year-old balding, enervated man finds both his hair and energy restored. A senior citizen recovers his interest in sex and reports his penis size has increased by 20%.

These are just some of the reports of people who claim to have been helped by supplemental doses of human growth hormone (HGH).

HGH is a hormone that is naturally present in the body when we are young, but which tends to disappear as we age. People who have taken HGH have found it produces striking improvements in their health, energy and sense of wellbeing. The list of benefits just seems to grow.

This now includes

- Younger skin
- Stronger bones
- Muscle gain without exercise
- Loss of body fat without dieting

- Less prone to sickness
- Faster wound healing
- More energy
- Enhanced sexual performance
- Stronger, healthier organs such as the liver, kidney, spleen
- Better exercise performance
- Lower blood pressure
- Fewer wrinkles
- Elimination of cellulite
- Better vision
- Improved mood
- Better memory.

WHAT IS HGH?

HGH is the mother of all hormones. It is a simple protein hormone released by the pituitary gland. It enters our blood-stream in bursts during sleep. It travels to the liver, where it is converted into a substance called insulin growth factor 1 (IGF1). IGF1 is the messenger molecule that travels to all parts of the body stimulating cell production and growth.

It is HGH that is responsible for telling our bodies to grow cells, bones, organs and muscles.

HGH is in plentiful supply until about age 20. Each decade from then on we lose approximately 20% of our HGH base level.

So, by the time you're 60 or 70, your body has access to only 15–20% of the HGH you had in your youth. HGH promotes growth by helping transport amino acids (the building blocks of protein) between cells and into cells. Amino acids are used by the body to create muscles and to build and restore organs, including the heart and skin.

Low levels of HGH cause ageing, because this hormone is primarily responsible for growth and regeneration of every cell in our bodies.

Every day, regardless of our age, millions of cells die and millions more new cells are produced. When we are young and growing, the high level of HGH causes our bodies to produce more new cells than those that die off. Our bodies expand in size and look young and fit.

As we get older, less HGH is produced (much of this decline can be attributed to our lifestyles), reversing the balance of new to old – more cells are dying than are being produced in every muscle, organ and part of our bodies. It's no wonder our body begins to break down.

This is why we become less functional and begin to age.

Indeed, the correct HGH levels are the secret to maintaining youth. Correct and specifically tailored exercise, diet, meditation and nutritional supplements will all naturally increase HGH and prolong youth. But, from around 50–60 years, even those treatments are not enough. It is the firm belief of most Anti-ageing physicians that to stay young many older people should supplement these treatments by taking HGH directly.

The evidence is extremely strong that they are right, in fact more than 28,000 different studies on HGH indicate that human growth hormone supplementation is indeed one secret to youth.

The first great controlled, random, double-blind (and therefore super-accurate) clinical study in this area was undertaken by Dr Daniel Rudman at the Medical College of Wisconsin, and was published in the prestigious New England Journal of Medicine in 1990.

Rudman treated 12 men aged 61 to 81 with HGH supplementation. The results were staggering. They actually reversed their body's ageing clocks.

Dr Rudman wrote: 'The effects of six months of human growth hormone on lean body mass and adipose-tissue mass were equivalent in magnitude to the changes incurred during 10–20 years of ageing.'

In interviews, the men reported incredible changes. One grey-haired 65-year-old found that his hair was turning black again. The wife of another man had trouble keeping up with her newly energised husband even though she was 15 years younger. A third man saw the wrinkles disappear on his face and hands.

Following up on his first test, Dr Rudman found that 26 other elderly men regrew their livers, spleens and muscles that had shrunk with age back to their youthful sizes.

These tests opened the floodgates in the scientific world and subsequently thousands more tests have verified Rudman's initial results.

For instance, in 1992 medical researchers at the renowned Stanford University stated: 'It is possible that physiological hormone replacement might reverse or prevent some of the 'inevitable' sequelae of ageing.'

Dr Julian Whitaker, of the Whitaker Health Institute in California, has been prescribing HGH to his patients. In his view, HGH is most effective in combating the effects of chronic disease that involve muscle wasting: stroke, chronic heart disease and AIDS. He feel it can even be beneficial in treating burns and in helping patients recover from surgery.

Dr Bengt-Ake Bengtsson, of Gothenberg, Sweden, states that the effects of 6 months of HGH therapy on lean body mass and fatty tissue was equivalent to reversing the ageing process by 10–20 years.

Dr Rudman does not believe HGH therapy will make people live longer, but that it will improve the quality of their life – stronger bones and muscles will improve mobility and independence, and mean fewer falls and broken bones.

And in 1989 Dr Franco Salomon at St Thomas Hospital in London began testing HGH on adults who had their pituitary gland removed due to tumours. The experiment lasted 6 months, at the end of which patients had averaged a 12 pound gain in muscle and a 12 pound fat loss, with lower serum cholesterol.

HGH LIMITS AND SIDE-EFFECTS

HGH can only be prescribed by a doctor, like any other hormonal treatment.

It has been reported to cause carpal tunnel syndrome and arthritis, and cause the growth of pre-cancerous cells. It has also been linked to water retention. Some men whose hormonal activity has been reawakened by HGH supplements find themselves growing small breasts. Finally, long-term HGH use in higher than physiological amounts has been known to cause the enlargement of bones of the hand, head and feet.

However, HGH for Anti-ageing purposes is prescribed in small, regular doses, to mimic the body's own natural secretions, which doctors have discovered cuts out most of the risks associated with its use in larger amounts. And recent studies have indicated that most, if not all, the undesirable side-effects are reversed when the patient stops taking HGH or the doses are reduced.

Normally healthy young people under 40 should not be taking HGH.

IS IT EXPENSIVE?

Until fairly recently, HGH supplements were difficult and expensive to make. HGH had to be extracted from the pituitary gland of human cadavers, and treatments were expensive. As a result, HGH supplements were used only in the treatment of dwarfism.

In 1980, two drug companies found inexpensive ways to produced HGH in laboratories. However, it is still expensive and can cost $10,000–$20,000 per year.

These prices are expected to fall soon, because the 7-year monopoly held by Eli Lilly expires. Together with recent innovations this may drive the prices down.

HGH replacement is also not desirable for all, because it must be administered by daily injection, which many people do not like.

WHAT ARE THE ALTERNATIVES? NATURAL HGH RELEASERS

People who wish to include HGH in **The Anti-ageing Diet** because of all the positive benefits but are concerned about the side-effects have other options – producing higher level of their own natural HGH! This is possible by stimulating your body to secrete even greater levels on its own. This option is safe, inexpensive and most satisfying.

There are two ways this can be achieved and combining the two is most powerful:

1. High–intensity exercise (which we will cover in another chapter) such as weight training, sprinting, squash etc. Long–distance running does not seem to be effective.
2. Secretagogues or natural HGH releasers.

There are certain amino acids and nutrients which in the right quantities and combinations can trigger the release of HGH.

These are:

Arginine

Ornithine

Niacin

Tyrosine

Glutathione

Methionine

People have also had good results using somatomedin, a HGH-releasing hormone which costs only a fraction of HGH itself. Studies have also suggested that melatonin can increase the production of HGH.

All of this is incredible news. But remember, HGH therapy is just a part of **The Anti-ageing Diet**. Great improvements in youth enhancement can be achieved by many other methods outlined in this **Anti-ageing Diet** as well.

DHEA

A 20-year study revealed that DHEA-S levels were lower in men who died of coronary heart disease than in healthier men.

Dr Majewoka, of the Maryland National Institute on Drug Abuse, showed DHEA to be effective in improving short and long-term memory.

In a year-long study at UCLA, it was discovered that DHEA increased muscle mass in both men and women, and that men gained strength and lost fat.

Anti-ageing hormones have long had a kind of chicken-and-egg relationship. Do falling hormone levels cause ageing, or is it ageing that causes lower levels of hormones?

Either way, maintaining optimum hormone levels suggested on **The Anti-ageing Diet** have been shown by researchers to not only halt ageing but also to combat a wide variety of debilitating diseases and even reverse the process of ageing for some of the body's organs.

DHEA (dehyroepiandosterone) is one of the most abundant naturally occurring hormones and one that seems capable of producing the most dramatic results in the following areas:

- Enhancing the immune system
- Reducing the incidence of cancer, heart disease and osteoporosis
- Lowering blood cholesterol and improving liver function
- Stabilising blood sugar levels to prevent the onset of adult diabetes
- Assisting in weight and fat loss
- Controlling Alzheimer's, lupus, AIDS and chronic fatigue syndrome
- Treating herpes, menopause, depression, memory and learning problems
- Prolonging life expectancy.

DHEA is produced by the adrenal glands. The body uses it to produce the sex hormones of testosterone, oestrogen and progesterone as well as cortisol.

Like HGH, DHEA levels increase until the age of about 15, then begin to drop off sharply so that at 65 we're producing only 10–20% of the DHEA we produced at 20.

According to Dr Samuel Yen at the University of California San Diego, DHEA may help people age more gracefully.

When taking DHEA, 82% of women and 67% of men scored higher test ratings in their ability to cope with stress, their quality of sleep and general well-being.

Dr William Regelson at Virginia Commonwealth University agrees that if you want to maintain youthful levels of health you need to maintain youthful levels of DHEA.

Scientists now believe that a person's risk of cancer may be linked to their levels of DHEA. It has been shown that women who suffer from ovarian cancer have extremely low levels of DHEA, suggesting that this hormone helps to prevent this type of cancer.

DHEA encourages the production of testosterone in men, which theoretically exacerbates a prostate condition, therefore it is not recommended for men with enlarged prostates or in cases where prostate cancer is feared.

One 20-year study found that DHEA levels were far lower in men who died of heart disease than in healthy men. Certainly, DHEA levels seem to be a predictor of coronary heart disease. A 1986 study published in the New England Journal of Medicine measured DHEA levels in 242 men aged 59–79. It was found that men whose DHEA levels were 140mcg or higher (20-year-old DHEA ranges 300–500mcg per deciliter) were less than half as likely to die of heart disease.

In a study of people with Alzheimer's disease, DHEA levels were found to be abnormally low. Many scientists believe DHEA may play a key role in improving functioning of the brain tissue and reducing the symptoms of Alzheimer's.

What researchers are now discovering, is that menopause is also associated with low DHEA levels and subsequent reduced bone density in women. The ovaries produce their own DHEA and when this slows during menopause the adrenal glands cannot adequately take over. The resulting overall deficiency in DHEA may be why osteoporosis afflicts so many older women.

While about 10% of diabetics suffer from low insulin levels, 90% suffer from insulin resistance. Their bodies manufacture normal levels of insulin, but they have difficulty using it.

As a result, insulin-resistant diabetics (with excess insulin in their blood) tend to have low DHEA levels. These low levels tend to contribute to heart problems and to obesity, particularly later in life. Insulin stimulates an enzyme which destroys DHEA.

In a 1988 study, DHEA was given to five men of normal weight at a dose of 1600mg per day. After 28 days of treatment, four out of five reported an average body fat decrease of 31% with no overall weight change. Their fat loss had been balanced by a gain in muscle mass. Simultaneously, their LDL cholesterol levels dropped by 7.5%. This change in body fat to muscle ratio may be due to DHEA's ability to help expend energy rather than store it for further use.

In a study at the Institute of Hearmath in California, it was found that DHEA levels can be naturally increased by people practising stress management and by listening to relaxing music. The study showed a 100% increase in DHEA levels and a 23% decrease in the hormone cortisol (the stress hormone).

Oral contraceptives also have been shown to reduce

DHEA levels. It has been suggested that women taking the Pill should consider DHEA replacement to negate its depleting effects.

Considering all the above evidence, it would seem logical that restoring DHEA levels would help restore a biological condition of youth.

HOW TO TAKE DHEA ON YOUR ANTI-AGEING DIET

In the US, DHEA can be bought without prescription at the supermarket. In Australia, however, it has not been approved and is difficult to get. DHEA replacement is very inexpensive – a month's supply of 50mg tablets should cost as little as $30.

You must always seek supervision from your Anti-ageing doctor before using DHEA.

Suggested Anti-ageing Diet doses: 25–150mg per day.

It's best to start at the lower end of this spectrum and increase the doses if necessary. You should have your DHEA levels checked every 3 months, and it is important to supplement your diet with extra antioxidants while taking DHEA.

Taking too much DHEA could cause your body's own production (as low as it is) to reduce. So it is wise to take DHEA on alternate days.

NATURAL DHEA STIMULATORS

Wild yam is a precursor (this means it biologically converts) to DHEA. Wild yam can be bought in tablet form and may be taken to naturally boost DHEA levels. Although it is not as effective as DHEA, it can be taken where smaller doses of DHEA are required or where DHEA is difficult to obtain. Take 1 capsule 3 times a day or seek advice from your Anti-ageing specialist on these doses.

OESTROGEN AND PROGESTERONE

The multi-billion-dollar industry in female hormones still generates much controversy.

Some claim oestrogen with progesterone helps curb menopausal symptoms. Sceptics reply that hormone replacement therapy puts women at higher risk of uterine and ovarian cancer, among other side-effects.

Other doctors say that women can treat themselves with oestrogen creams and or natural sources of progesterone.

More and more research is providing strong evidence that taking oestrogen significantly reduces the death rate from **all** postmenopausal causes, including heart attack and stroke.

Approximately 300 different tissues are equipped with oestrogen receptors. This means that oestrogen can affect a wide range of tissues and organs, including the brain, liver, bones and skin. The uterus, urinary tract, breasts, skin and blood vessels also depend on oestrogen to stay toned and flexible.

Women's hormonal fluctuations play havoc with their systems, which may vary widely within a single day and drive you 'crazy'. A long-term decline in sex hormone levels produces symptoms such as drier skin, brittle hair, loss of libido, mood swings, hot flushes, night sweats, vaginal dryness and itching, ageing skin, increased chance of heart disease, osteoporosis, colon cancer and mental deterioration.

This usually begins around the age of 40, however, it can start by the early thirties.

Scientific studies and reports from numerous women show that oestrogen can ease or eliminate menopausal woes. In order to get the positive effects of oestrogen, doctors believe you have to take it for at least seven years, although 95% of women continue with this for three years or less.

When oestrogen treatments were first discovered, this hormone was usually prescribed alone. Only later doctors discovered that it was more effective and safer to use with progesterone.

Progesterone replacement, however, is not without its own controversy. The best form of progesterone replacement is natural hormone supplements. These, unfortunately, are hard to come by because drug companies cannot patent them and therefore are not interested in selling them commercially.

They produce a sythesised product called progestin which closely resembles natural progesterone. Doctors believe progestin has a long list of side-effects and exposes women to unnecessary risks, such as abnormal menstrual flow or cessation, fluid retention, nausea, insomnia, jaundice, depression, fever, weight fluctuations, allergic reactions and the development of male characteristics. Natural progesterone has few side-effects other than occasionally producing a feeling of euphoria.

Oestrogen therapy has come under controversy most notably for causing breast cancer. One study revealed patients on oestrogen (with and without progestin) had a 30–40% increased risk of breast cancer. Another study, however, reported no increased risk of cancer. These conflicting results underscore the continued uncertainty over oestrogen's role in breast cancer. For this reason, oestrogen treatment is not recommended for women with high risk of breast cancer.

The relationship between oestrogen and the risk of breast cancer has been studied intensively. At the present time there is no conclusive evidence that oestrogen doses prevent osteoporosis and cardiovascular disease or increase the risk of breast cancer, however, there is some evidence that the two hormones together can increase this risk by as much as 30%.

Doctors are still at odds about how seriously to take these reports. They say that HRT benefits outweigh the risks for most people. Eight times as many women die of heart attacks as die of breast cancer.

THE GOOD AND BAD SEX HORMONES

It is also important to realise that not all oestrogens are equivalent in their action on breast tissue, and may explain some of this controversy.

Natural oestrogen takes 3 forms:

Estrotone

Estradiol

Estriol

Estrotone is the most stimulating to breast tissue with estriol the least. Estriol has actually been shown to decrease the risk of breast cancer.

Synthetic oestrogen supplements, however, seem to exclude estriol, and are composed primarily of the other two, yet natural oestrogen is high in estriol.

THE ANTI-CANCER HORMONE

Women with breast cancer have been shown in one study to excrete 30–60% less estriol than non-cancer patients and higher remission rates of cancer occurred in those whose estriol levels rose. Therefore, low levels of estriol relative to estradiol and estrotone correlate with an increased risk of breast cancer.

This example illustrates how complicated the biology of the body really is. Will oestrogen therapy increase a woman's chances of developing breast cancer? Conflicting evidence has kept this controversy alive, but the risk appears to be small, weighed against the long-term benefit for heart and bones.

Although many women take oestrogen supplements, many also report feeling worried, sceptical or discouraged about it. It seems from research that one-fifth of women given a prescription for oestrogen never fill it. Of the other 80%, one-third stop taking the supplement within nine months and more than half stop within a year.

HRT AND THE ANTI-AGEING DIET

Natural supplements listed below may be the solution for many women, however, these are not nearly as powerful as hormone supplements.

Women may benefit from a more holistic approach suggested as part of your **Anti-ageing Diet**, such as the avoidance of smoking and excessive alcohol, more aerobic exercise, a low-fat, high-fibre diet and vitamin and mineral supplements. Indeed, women have reported that menopausal symptoms eased or disappeared as they paid more attention to their exercise and diet.

Taking vitamins such as beta-carotene and Vitamin E can raise progesterone levels. Natural sources of both oestrogen and progesterone are found in soybean, tofu, miso and soy milk. These products contain phytoestrogens. Phytoestrogen supplements are also an alternative to synthetic oestrogens. Women who want could try natural oestrogen extracted from wild yam.

Other botanical nutrients that can help ease menopausal systems are:

- Black Cohosh
- Dong Quai
- Motherwort
- Liquorice root
- Red raspberry

TESTOSTERONE

After puberty, testosterone levels drop gradually in men. If this fall is more dramatic, due to injury or infection, it could result in a condition known as hypogonadism.

Some sure signs of low testosterone levels are loss of sex drive, impotence, fatigue, irritability, depression, joint aches, dry skin, osteoporosis, weight loss.

Testosterone levels are affected by a number of external factors such as illness, medications, psychological states, obesity, exercise, lifestyle ie smoking and drinking. Other factors, such as nutritional deficiency, diabetes and low HGH, may contribute to lower testosterone levels.

Men diagnosed with hypogonadism are good candidates for testosterone replacement therapy (TRT).

One study of men over 50 who received TRT found

that it renewed strength, improved balance, increased red blood cell count, increased libido and lowered LDL cholesterol.

Dr Michael Perring, medical director of Optimal Health Clinic in London, believes that TRT in conjunction with DHEA is beneficial to men with low testosterone levels for their age. Numerous studies have also shown the link between low testosterone and high risks of cardiovascular disease.

Advocates of HGH therapy are also focusing on TRT because of its relative cost and bone-strengthening qualities.

TESTOSTERONE ON YOUR ANTI-AGEING DIET

If you have hypogonadism or below-optimal testosterone levels, we recommend only natural testosterone, because synthetic products are linked to liver damage. If you are considering TRT you must be aware of both the risks and benefits. The largest concern is TRT's potential to stimulate prostate cancer and reduce HDL cholesterol.

Using a precursor such as DHEA is the safest way to stimulate higher testosterone levels. Should you be considering TRT at all, it is important to undergo a full assessment, including full blood and other serum level checks, by a qualified Anti-ageing doctor before undertaking any supplementation or treatment.

MELATONIN

Imagine a 'wonder drug' that extended your lifespan by 25% or more. Imagine, too, that this drug not only extended your life but maintained your youth, enabling you to enjoy work, sex and social activities with the same zest and vigour that marked your life at 45. Imagine, finally, that this drug had no harmful side-effects or long-term dangers, because it is not actually a drug at all, but a substance that occurs naturally in your body.

The fact is, we don't have to imagine that at all. It already exists in every living substance from algae to humans. It is called *melatonin*.

Melatonin is produced by the pineal gland and research has revealed some amazing outcomes:

Researchers at Tulane University School of Medicine in New Orleans have studies that suggest melatonin can stop or retard the advance of human breast cancer cells.

A 1995 study by an Italian researcher demonstrated that melatonin boosted the immune system of people under extreme stress.

Melatonin helps prevent heart disease by lowering blood cholesterol, combats AIDS, Alzheimer's, Parkinson's, asthma, diabetes and cataracts.

It has also been found to be effective in re-setting the biological clocks of travellers moving across time zones and is a natural sleeping pill inducing sleep without the side-effects of sedatives.

In addition, it has been shown to be a powerful anti-oxidant, helping to keep the body young.

The main function of the pineal gland is to help govern our biological rhythms (circadian rhythms) that take place over the day, such as the sleep-wake cycle. It also governs seasonal rhythms. Researchers see this gland and hormone as a kind of orchestra conductor, coordinating and controlling our other hormone-release and immune responses. The pineal gland communicates with these other system through its messenger, melatonin.

Changes in melatonin set off a range of responses, such as puberty, menstruation and sleep. It also alerts our bodies to produce antibodies to combat disease.

So, you can see how important the presence and maintenance of correct level of this hormone are for the optimal functioning of our bodies throughout our life.

As we've seen, nature isn't much interested in us after we've gotten too old to reproduce. Our pineal gland is our internal clock that 'knows' how old we are and when we are past our prime. It responds by producing lower levels of melatonin, signalling our other systems to break down, causing us to age.

What if we could somehow raise our levels of melatonin after they start to fall? What if for the rest of our lives we could duplicate the levels of melatonin we had in our youth? We would in effect be 'tricking' our bodies into believing they are still young, giving orders to produce higher levels of sex hormones and a well-functioning immune system to fight off disease ... chronologically we would be old, yet biologically we would still be young.

Researchers have found that melatonin supplementation helps the body mimic a youthful state. Not only that, but melatonin helps strengthen our immune systems, prevents cancer and improves sexual functioning.

One of the ways melatonin helps combat cancer is as a powerful antioxidant. It is the only antioxidant capable of penetrating every cell of the body and is the most active and effective of all naturally occurring compounds.

For example, in certain tests melatonin proved to be five times more powerful than glutathione and at least twice as effective as powerful Vitamin E. Furthermore, most anti-oxidants are either water-soluble or fat-soluble. Melatonin is making it a wider-ranging antioxidant than its vitamin or mineral counterparts.

MELATONIN ON YOUR ANTI-AGEING DIET

With melatonin, remember less is more. Although melatonin plays an extremely important role in our bodies, it is present in only tiny amounts, even at our youthful peak. Larger doses of melatonin won't help. Children should not take melatonin and people with auto-immune disorders, leukemia or lymphoma should consult an Anti-ageing doctor before use. Pregnant or nursing mothers also should avoid melatonin. On the other hand, women on HRT should take melatonin without fear of any ill-effects.

As melatonin drops most sharply around age 45, melatonin supplementation should begin around then and not before, except for short-term use, such as jet lag. People with a family history of cancer or cardiovascular disease might begin in their late 30s. The idea is to start taking melatonin when your levels drop off and not before, because extra melatonin (above your optimal physiological needs) will not benefit you.

Remember, always take melatonin at bed time as it generally makes you sleepy, so it should not be taken before you drive or operate machinery.

Melatonin is hard to get in Australia, however, it is freely available on supermarket shelves in the US. The synthetic form is better than that which is made from animals because this eliminates the risk of contamination.

Remember, each person's physiology is unique so it is advisable to get your melatonin level checked at your Anti-ageing centre. Melatonin in the range 0.5mg–12 mg is usually effective. It's best to start on low doses such as 1–2mg and increase this if you find it does not help. Reduce your doses if you find you are waking up tired and groggy. It is wise to take melatonin every second day, because it is not yet known whether it can inhibit natural production. Taken on a full stomach it may also be less effective.

Note: Most long-term studies conducted on melatonin have been done on animals and are yet to be conclusively shown to work on humans. The only proven safe use is as a short-term remedy for jet lag and sleep disorder.

THYROID HORMONES (TH)

The thyroid has tremendous responsibilities and affects all metabolic activity. It regulates temperature, heart rate and metabolism. If your thyroid isn't functioning optimally neither are you.

Some of the following symptoms sound just like old age and are tolerated as such, yet many of these are as a direct result of thyroid deficiencies: Fatigue, weakness, frequent colds and respiratory ailments, laboured breathing, muscle cramps, persistent lower back pain, common bruising, poor memory, headaches, emotional instability, anxiousness, cold hands and feet, dry skin, coarse hair or hair loss, stiff joints, loss of appetite, reduced interest in sex, clogged arteries, weak heart and circulation.

Of course, these symptom may be from ageing but they are far more likely to be from a combination of low TH and nutritional deficiencies.

Correcting this condition can quickly reverse many of these ailments.

Dr Murry Isreal was called to see a patient who was so debilitated that a priest had been called to give her last rites. Examination had shown her breathing was shallow, heart beat faint, blood pressure dangerously low, coronary arteries clogged, her hair was totally white and skin was marked by dead patches.

Dr Israel administered 10mg of TH brewer's yeast (rich in B vitamins) three times a day. Within two weeks, the woman was mentally alert and strong enough to walk to church. Her dead skin had peeled off, leaving her with a smooth, pink complexion, and some black reappeared in her hair. She lived an active life for another 20 years.

This is a clear example of how hormone replacement with vitamin supplements has, in effect, reversed the ageing process.

THYROID HORMONES AND YOUR ANTI-AGEING DIET

TH deficiency needs to be correctly diagnosed, and you should have your levels regularly checked, even if you feel well, as part of your **Anti-ageing** Diet regime.

The following TH cofactors and thyroid gland stimulators will help improve the proper functioning of your thyroid.

L-Tyrosine	500mg twice a day with B6
Sea kelp	as directed on label
Raw thyroid	
Glandular	as directed by doctor
Vitamin B complex	100mg with meals

With riboflavin	50mg twice daily
Brewer's yeast	as directed on label
Iron chelate	as directed on label
Vitamin A	15000IU
Plus beta-carotene	
Vitamin C	500mg 4 times per day
Vitamin E	400UI daily
Zinc	50mg daily

Section 9

STRESS ON THE ANTI-AGEING DIET

I n **The Anti-ageing Diet** we have looked at the ageing process as a result of deteriorating biochemistry, and factors that contribute to it.

We have included a poor diet, exposure to pollution and toxins, a sedentary lifestyle, heavy consumption of alcohol, smoking etc.

We've explored a range of nutritional supplements, lifestyle choices and hormonal treatments that can slow, ease and reverse the ageing process.

Yet perhaps the most powerful Anti-ageing weapon you have at your disposal is your mind.

Your health is greatly affected by how you react to stressful events – setbacks, deadlines, conflicts and losses.

One of the biggest factors that affect lifespan and the ageing process is stress. In this modern age it is almost impossible to live a stress-free life.

Learning to change how you react to situations, learning relaxation techniques, learning to meditate and generally committing to a positive, open attitude to life can help keep you years younger, reducing your biological age.

Remember, it is not stress that directly harms us, but distress. Distress occurs when we experience prolonged emotional stress and don't or are not able to deal with it in a positive manner.

Our bodies react to stress in 3 phases, outlined by Dr Hans Selye.

1. Alarm
2. Resistance
3. Exhaustion

The alarm phase is the well-known 'fight-or-flight' response. Your body releases a hormone called cortisol as it prepares to do battle. However, since modern day stressors are not physical things we can generally turn and fight or run away from, the alarm stage is lengthened, leading us into the next phase, resistance, and then exhaustion.

It is during exhaustion that the body becomes distressed and the outcome of this ranges from fatigue to disease and death.

HOW TO LIVE WITH STRESS

Stress itself is not a negative thing. It is our response to stress which is negative. This gives us some control over the stress even if we cannot control the thing that causes stress. We can control our response to it, which is more important!

People who truly understand this have a great advantage in life. The power of choice and the degree to which we feel we have control over our lives in an increasingly uncertain world is the degree to which we have the ability to control stress and everything else in our lives, too.

That is why this concept of our right to choose to have control over our lives is central to the theme of many self-help teachers and writers.

The one major difference between humans and farm animals is our ability to make a choice. Unfortunately, not enough of us exercise our right to make a choice and take control of our lives.

Many of us take on a victim's mentality when things do not go right for us and give up control by feeling helpless and oppressed, rather than changing our reaction through making a different choice on how we feel about what has occurred.

If you do not have the confidence to accept that you have a choice and just let stress happen to you, by not taking the right action, your body will probably respond with anxiety, headaches, stomach ache, ulcers, depression, allergies and heart disease. If left unchecked, in the long run, negative responses to stress will cause a lowering of your immune system, potentially leading to cancer and other diseases traditionally associated with ageing.

In response to a stressful situation our body produces 'stress hormones' – cortisol, epinephrine and norepinephrine. These set off a chain reaction resulting in higher levels of free radicals. Elevated levels of cortisol are also associated with acne, obesity, alcoholism, Alzheimer's, Parkinson's, multiple sclerosis, psoriasis, arthritis and many more.

25 ANTI-AGEING DIET STRATEGIES FOR DEALING WITH STRESS

1. Go to an Anti-ageing specialist for a check up
2. Take a siesta
3. Don't take on other people's problems
4. Spend quality time with friends
5. Become more spiritual
6. Adopt a pet

7. Take up a hobby
8. Learn to prioritise
9. Live in a calm, beautiful environment
10. Learn to look for positives in every negative situation
11. Control your finances well
12. Practise meditation
13. Smile more
14. Improve your communication skills
15. Exercise more
16. Change your diet
17. Cut back on alcohol
18. Cut out caffeine
19. Stop smoking
20. Try to keep things in perspective
21. Get a massage
22. Don't dwell in the past or on mistakes or failures
23. Take B group vitamins, St John's wort and glutamine
24. Learn to express your anger positively and respectfully
25. Don't take setbacks personally

HOW TO BEAT STRESS

Meditation is one of the most powerful forms of stress relief, mind development and relaxation. With the aid of meditation, it has been proven that stress levels drop dramatically and assist in creating a more relaxed, less anxious, more centred and peaceful frame of mind.

There are many different forms of meditation, but no matter what type of meditation you practise or prefer, they all have the same goal – stillness of the mind.

Meditation is not a state of sleep, it is a low-consciousness waking, in which the mind is calm, yet still.

During successful meditative states, muscles relax, metabolism slows, breathing and heart rate are lowered and blood flow to the brain increases.

Daily meditation seems to have the long-term benefit of lowering anxiety, improving mental functioning and lowering your biological age.

According to Dr Keith Wallace's study of meditators, people who meditated for more than five years had biological ages averaging 12 years younger than a control group who did not meditate.

In the past, meditation for some people has been difficult – not being able to 'switch off', inability to visualise or even not knowing what to do. These are just some of the reasons people do not benefit from the power of meditation.

There is now audio meditation technology that will give you all the benefits of meditation without having to consciously work at it.

Holosync® audio technology is a scientifically developed audio program that safely and effortlessly allows you to experience deep meditation and accelerate your mental and spiritual growth. The technology is placed on cassette tape beneath soothing music and environmental sounds and is a most powerful personal growth and mind development tool. Listening to the cassette transports you to a deep, peaceful, highly pleasurable and relaxing state of meditation.

You are able to experience deep meditation, dramatic increases in the production of a whole variety of beneficial brain chemicals, including pleasure-causing endorphins, as well as a number of others proven to slow ageing and increase longevity and well-being.

Regular use will allow your stress levels to drop and

enhance your ability to deal calmly and clearly with whatever comes at you from the world.

Your learning ability will increase; creativity goes up, intuition increases, focus and concentration increases and personal self-awareness increases. Achievement becomes easier, and without the same feelings of anxiety and stress.

By stimulating your brain with meditation you can expect:

- Greatly improved mental abilities
- Dramatic reduction in stress and anxiety
- Improved health
- A new sense of mental, emotional and physical balance and well-being
- Heightened creativity and problem-solving ability
- Increased focus, concentration and learning ability
- Enhanced memory
- Increased motivation and confidence
- Production in the brain of many vital neurochemicals proven to slow ageing and keep the body young, alive and fully functioning
- Better, more restful sleep
- More happiness and 'flow' in your life
- Elimination of unresolved mental and emotional blocks

ANTI-AGEING EXERCISE FOR THE BRAIN

Just as we exercise our bodies to feel better and improve our physical health, stimulating the brain in this manner 'exercises' the brain, bringing better mental and emotional health and increased intellectual functioning. Furthermore, the long-term effects of regular use can possibly delay for decades the deterioration of the brain traditionally associated with ageing.

Scientists have found that the brain releases many highly beneficial substances, including HGH (human growth hormone), which we ordinarily make in decreasing quantities as we get older, resulting in many ageing symptoms including loss of muscle tone, increased weight gain, loss of stamina and many diseases associated with ageing.

You can help to stimulate the production of HGH and other beneficial substances in the brain, easily and safely, by exposing yourself each day to meditation.

Recent research shows that meditation dramatically lowers levels of the main stress-inducing hormone in the body and increases levels of the hormone that is your main buffer against stress. It also dramatically affects production of three important hormones related to both increased longevity and enhanced well-being – cortisol, DHEA and melatonin.

Cortisol is a hormone naturally produced by the adrenal glands. It is the major age-accelerating hormone in the brain and it interferes with learning and memory and is in general bad news for your health and well-being. It is also the 'stress' hormone – the more you have, the more stressed you feel, the more susceptible you are to disease and the faster you age.

DHEA is also produced by the adrenal glands. DHEA levels are a key determinant of physiological age and resistance to disease. When levels are low, you are more susceptible to ageing and disease. When they are high the body is at its peak – vibrant, healthy and able to combat disease effectively. DHEA acts as a buffer against stress-related hormones (such as cortisol), which is why as you get older and make less you are more susceptible to stress and disease.

Melatonin is a hormone that helps to create restful sleep. We make less of it as we age, and since during sleep many important rejuvenation substances are created in the brain, the inability to sleep soundly can dramatically decrease the quality of your life and greatly accelerate the ageing process.

BEATING STRESS ON YOUR ANTI-AGEING DIET

Meditate daily using any form of meditation that you find comfortable and which works for you.

Get regular massages, weekly if you can afford it.

Take supplements of glutamine, Vitamin B group, especially B5, and St John's wort.

The best and most effective way to stay young and live a full and happy life is to ensure you have a well balanced life, taking time in the day for pleasure, achievement and obligation. Fill your life with a wide variety of challenges and joy that will nourish your mind, body and spirit. Listen to yourself, discover what you need and find a self-fulfilling way to achieve it.

STRESS AND FATIGUE

Technology over the past decade has increased to a point where our man-made, wired-up world has taken over our natural world. Some scientists estimate that you are now daily exposed to 100 million times the electromagnetic frequency radiation your grandparents experienced.

EMF disrupts your natural energy levels, triggering stress responses. Both alternative and traditional doctors report that

EMF is a co-factor in increasing your daily stress levels. Stress can impair your body's natural ability to heal. It adds even more stress to your own stress and fatigue, and to your already-taxed system. EMF is generated from computers, mobile phones, air travel, office and household appliances which all contribute to energy depletion and increasing fatigue.

This can cause a variety of symptoms such as headaches, fatigue, muscle tension, personal stress, mood swings, impaired mental concentration and focus, increased emotional volatility, depression, feelings of jet lag, sleep deprivation, loss of momentum, and diminished responses to cope with the demands of life.

EMF' has been linked to a wide range of diseases and disorders, including weakening of the immune, nervous and muscular systems, cancer, breast cancer, increased stress, Alzheimer's, anxiety and depression. EMF' is also said to be a cause of a condition known as electrical sensitivity syndrome, whose symptoms are similar to those of chronic fatigue syndrome, symptoms which the working public report, due to the rapidly expanding technology of the world.

This problem has been categorised as a new form of pollution as consequential as air and water pollution. It has also been likened to the discovered hazards of asbestos and cigarette smoking. In terms of its cumulative health effects, it's been compared to the slow process of lead poisoning. It is a problem that is growing rapidly – and at a compounding rate. Fortunately, public awareness of EMF is also growing.

'Electromagnetic pollution may be the most significant form of pollution man has produced in this century. All the more dangerous because it is invisible and insensible.' – **Andrew Weil, MD**

What can be done about this problem? Not much, one would think, except turn off the electricity. In this day and age that is not an option. There is, however, an electro-magnetic deflector product you can obtain that is shown to reduce stress levels by 30% to 70%, especially stress caused by EMF sources such as computers and mobile phones. *(for more information see appendix)*

Section 10

EXERCISE ON THE ANTI-AGEING DIET
By John Gearon

EXERCISE IS NOT AN OPTION ANYMORE: IT'S NECESSARY AND FUN

Exercise. The mere word brings fear into the hearts of many people.

And I can understand why.

It's time-consuming, it's painful and it zaps your energy.

But this is only short term. In the long term, regular exercise is easy, painless and fun and a necessity as part of your **Anti-ageing Diet**, to give you the health, energy and youth you are looking for.

In order to succeed at doing exercise, there are a few fundamental things you should be aware of:

- Exercise is not something you do only once. In order to get the benefits of exercise this must become part of your life. If you want to keep your teeth strong and healthy you need to brush and floss twice each day. Exercise is of equal importance, to keep your body strong, flexible and active.
- Exercise needs to become a daily habit. I believe it is easier to do exercise each day than it is every second

day or twice a week. This is because we are creatures of habit, and if we make exercise a daily habit, after a short while we don't even have to think about it or try to fit it in, it just seems to find a time and place in our day.

I DON'T HAVE TIME FOR EXERCISE – I'M TOO BUSY!

This has to be the number one excuse people make for not doing exercise. And for many people, it is true. Today, people live incredibly demanding lives and are 'time poor'. Juggling multiple demands on your time can be difficult, draining and exhausting.

This is exactly why you need to do exercise. Apart from the many other health benefits of exercise on **The Anti-ageing Diet**, it gives you more energy to deal with these demands.

IT COMES DOWN TO TIME MANAGEMENT . . . OR DOES IT?

In order to succeed on your **Anti-ageing Diet**, you need 4 very important ingredients.

1. Commitment
2. Goals
3. Determination
4. Willingness to re-prioritise

YOU DO NOT NEED WILLPOWER, NOR MORE TIME TO FIT EVERYTHING IN

Everybody has the same 24 hours a day. So ask yourself: how is it that some people do manage to fit it all in when they are doing whatever you're doing and more?

It's simple!

They do these 4 things. They make a commitment, they set clear, effective goals, they have the determination (ie they want to achieve their goals badly enough), and they have a willingness to re-prioritise.

Without these 4 critical factors, you may find yourself finding reasons why you cannot do exercise, instead of finding reasons why you can and must.

Once you make a commitment, you will be amazed at what will happen to you, your time and most importantly your self-esteem.

Here's another little secret for you . . . There is no such thing as *time management*. Think about it.

How can you manage time when there are so many unknown things that just seem to pop up in your day to take up (or waste) your time.

Everybody has heard of or read Stephen Covey's Book *The 7 Habits of Highly Effective People*. But fewer have read his book *First Thing First* (which, by the way, is one of his 7 habits).

What this book says in summary is that you should not follow the clock. Instead, you should follow the compass.

What this means is that you shouldn't try to fit everything into your day. Simply decide what is most important to you and do those things first. Everything else can wait or be left undone, because we cannot do everything in life.

It's all a matter of importance and priorities. Each day you must continually attend to and re-adjust your priorities as necessary.

But I promise you, if you make a commitment to exercise as a lifestyle and daily priority, you will not miss out on anything and will still find time and have more energy to fit all the other things in.

There is another great teacher – Dr Fred Gross – who I have been lucky enough to hear speak. His message is also very important to you, and it's very simple. Stop and look at your day. Evaluate everything you did and who you spent time with. Now, decide if that was time-efficient or necessary. You will be amazed at how many time-wasters in your day you have the option to eliminate. This time could equally have been replaced with doing exercise.

WHAT ABOUT MULTI-TASKING?

Another great way to find time in your day is to multi-task – do two things at once.

Find activities or things in your day that you can do while exercising. A friend of mine used to catch a bus to work in the morning. In peak hour it took him 35 minutes. Now he runs to work and it takes him 40 minutes. Incorporating exercise into his life he only needed to find 5 more minutes. This may not be possible for you, however, I am certain there are other options available to you to multi-task.

MAKE AN APPOINTMENT WITH YOURSELF

This is another great way to ensure you build exercise into your daily life. Open your diary and pretend someone has called you to make an appointment with them. Write that 1/2 or 1 hour into your diary (if you are really busy you might want to do this daily for weeks in advance). Then when other business or pressing matters come up, you simply schedule it around those appointments. You will be amazed to find you now have a time hole in your diary for you to go and do your exercise without fail.

HOW TO LOVE EXERCISE EVEN MORE

One of the most effective ways to learn to love exercise is to focus on the result that you want to achieve – either fat burning or muscle conditioning.

So many people exercise and resent it because they associate a strict exercise regime with punishment to compensate for things they enjoy more.

Instead, exercise should be looked at as one of the ways of pampering and caring for one's self. Once you focus on how the benefits from your workout are really going to enhance how you feel for the rest of the day, you will find that you start to love it and look forward to it a lot more. You begin to feel as if you have given yourself a treat.

What people generally do when they commence any type of exercise, and most certainly when in a weight-training regime, is monitor what they did in their last training session and continually try to top their last workout.

For example, if they are doing a resistance-training exercise, they focus on a certain amount of repetitions and sets with the appropriate weight in excess of what they did at their last workout.

They are educated that their workout is a success only if they match or exceed the last workout. This isn't a reasonable or smart way to measure one's progress. They fail to take into consideration what has happened since their last workout, whether they have been getting optimum nutrition, rest, or whether or not their body has recovered from the last workout.

The most effective way to stay motivated and avoid the physiological emotional roller coaster of ups and downs is not to count the reps or weights during your workout, but assess how you are honestly feeling compared to your last training session.

Be aware of what has happened in between workouts. Focus on training with the weight that you want and with each training set go to the maximum degree of effort. That's the point where you cannot do another repetition.

DON'T COUNT REPS, JUST ENJOY THE PROCESS

Most people get in there and count the reps and weight, not focusing on getting the best stimulus for maximum results. It's exactly the same with other exercises. Focus only on your heart rate, not the levels displaying your progress as with bikes, treadmills and other machines. Being honest about how you feel is the most effective way to monitor progress.

You don't drive your car and just look at the speed your are doing. You also notice the rpm on the motor. If the next time you drove your car you noticed that the speed was the same but your revs were up quite considerably, you would think there is something wrong with the motor. Have respect for your body like you do your car.

If you are training at a consistent level of intensity, yet your heart rate is in excess of what it normally is, that is a true sign of over-exercising and proof that you haven't recovered from your last exercise session.

It will certainly reduce your level of enjoyment, leading to a loss of motivation to return to do another workout.

Another way to really look at loving exercise is to perceive it as the one part of the day when you are truly doing something for yourself, physically and emotionally.

THE BEST EXERCISE FOR A LONG LIFE

One of the most effective exercises for longevity is walking. Walking actually gets the whole system happening, flushing out toxins and waste and burning your fat stores.

Swimming is another. It is non-weight-bearing – a phenomenal exercise that combines the upper and lower body.

Swimming is also great for the calming, soothing effects of the water, and the mental switch off that can be achieved due of the lack of external influences.

Resistance training or other physical activity also helps increase longevity. When people who are retired take up a physical activity like gardening etc they admit to feeling better than they have for years.

Previously, their lifestyle was usually very sedentary. We must get back into natural physical activity, which our body is designed for.

The Industrial Age perhaps saves us time, but it is also

killing us off through technology, equipment, motor vehicles, and all of the other labour-saving activities. With the time saved by these conveniences, we should be incorporating exercises and other physical activities that will promote well-being, and assist in promoting the quality of our lives now and in later years. If we do not look after our body now *where else are we going to live?*

THE ANTI-AGEING DIET'S APPROACH TO EXERCISE

There is a simple 3-pillar approach to Anti-ageing exercise. Each week your exercise programs should include all these three to be most effective. We'll talk about all of these below:

- Pillar One – Fat Burning – for optimal muscle & fat balance.
- Pillar Two – Cardiovascular Fitness – Heart & Lungs Conditioning.
- Pillar Three – Muscle-Strength Conditioning – Physical Structure.

NOW IS A GREAT TIME TO GET FIT

Exercise must be fun or else you won't stick with it. One way to keep exercise fun is to keep exercise as safe and as effective as possible. Injury or muscle soreness will quickly destroy your enthusiasm. Exercise right each time and you are more likely to stick with it and see good results at last.

Remember to always warm up and cool down whenever

exercising. Warming up will also bring your body from its normal passive level of activity to being in a state prepared to begin exercise by increasing the blood flow to your muscles.

Warm ups should be done at a very low intensity, in order to prepare your body for exercise. You should cool down with stretching for at least 10 minutes after exercise by decreasing your exercise level to help your cardiovascular system to return to its normal level and balance your system.

GREAT EXERCISE REVOLVES AROUND JUST A FEW THINGS

- **Frequency**. To improve your cardiovascular fitness, you should exercise a minimum of three times a week. To burn fat, you should exercise at least four times a week, for longer duration, at a lower intensity.
- **Intensity** refers to burning body fat or burning sugars. This is how hard you work out. You must work out your rate of perceived exertion in proportion to your theoretic maximum heart rate. This is done by calculating 220 minus your age, and your intensity level is to then work within certain percentages of this number, which is referred to as the heart-rate zoning section. (see below)
- **Duration** refers to the number of minutes you exercise in each workout session. To maximise the benefit of your workout program it is important that you exercise at least 20 minutes per session to achieve your cardiovascular goals, and optimally around 40 minutes to achieve your body-fat-burning goals.

TRAINING SHOULD BE EASY AND FUN

If you are new to exercising, use a heart-rate training zone of no greater than 60-75% (of your maximum heart rate of 220 less your age), which is your body-fat-burning zone, for the first few weeks of your exercise program.

You may even need to start at or below 50% and work up to it gradually as your body starts to adapt to the exercise.

As your fitness levels improve, re-calculate your heart-rate zone up to conducting your sessions between 70 and 85%, as long as you can maintain intensity for a minimum of 20 minutes. This is purely to work on your sugar burning and condition your cardiovascular fitness.

The majority of your workouts should be done at the lower end of intensity, which is between 60 and 75%, to optimally burn body fat, and to flush your system of toxins to achieve optimum health and wellness.

You should never exceed the intensity of 85% of your theoretical maximum heart rate. There are no significant gains in cardiovascular fitness at such a high level of intensity, but there is a significantly higher risk of injury.

BURNING FATS, NOT SUGAR

Research shows that exercising within a specific heart-rate range is the optimum way to both monitor your exercise intensity and achieve maximum results to burn fat or burn sugar.

Example of Fat-Burning & Sugar-Burning Heart-Rate Training Zones for a 40-year-old.

Theoretical Maximum Heart Rate is 220 beats per minute (BPM) 220 − 40 (age) = 180 BPM

Fat Burning – Heart-Rate Zone between 60 to 75% of Maximum Heart Rate

Multiple 180 × 60% = 108 BPM – Low End
Multiple 180 × 75% = 135 BPM – High End

Sugar Burning – Heart-Rate Zone between 75 to 85% of Maximum Heart Rate

Multiple 180 × 75% = 135 BPM – Low End
Multiple 180 × 85% = 153 BPM – High End

If your primary goal is to burn fat you should exercise at a level between 60 and 75% of your theoretical maximum heart rate, as outlined in the example above. If your goal is to improve your cardiovascular fitness and sugar burning, then you should exercise at 75% to 85% of your maximum heart rate.

The key to get most optimum fat burning is to stay within your fat-burning zone. Most people still hold to the old belief 'go hard or go home' or 'no pain no gain', which is OK to some extent, for an elite athlete.

As for the rest of us, to train at that intensity indefinitely will only turn us off exercise because it is too uncomfortable. At such levels, the body breaks down or gets sick, either due to injury or because of susceptibility to virus and or infections. This occurs because training at such a high level of intensity leads the body to be burning lots of sugar as well as producing excess lactate acid, which increases the acidity of your biological terrain (blood, urine and saliva).

For the majority of the population, their goal is to burn

stored body fat. The most effective way to monitor this is by your heart rate, using one of the many heart-rate-monitoring watches and chest-strap systems on the market.

The other way to evaluate your fat-burning and sugar-burning perimeter is to monitor how you are feeling while exercising.

If your goal is to burn fat while exercising – a runner for example.

- You should still be able to talk comfortably while running.
- You should have a slight/moderate amount of perspiration.
- Your field of vision should still be wide and you can look around.
- You should be able to maintain your ability to take in information from your surroundings, colour, shapes etc.

If you are sugar burning while exercising – a runner for example.

- Cannot talk comfortably.
- Massive amounts of perspiration are excreted
- Field of vision becomes quite narrow and tunnelled.
- Information from your surroundings become less prominent, with less colour etc.

ARE YOU CRAVING SUGARS AFTER SOME WORKOUTS?

Our body isn't naturally comfortable burning sugar the whole time. It likes to keep a primary reserve of stored sugars. Remember, our origins are that of a primate being, which in olden times meant life was basically a matter of hunting or being hunted. Both of those activities require an intense degree of energy expenditure from the body to survive, purely a sugar-burning activity. When we exercise to the extent that we are burning sugars and depleting our sugar reserves, our body is feeling vulnerable and signals to us by way of cravings to replenish our empty sugar zones. This function of the body is an in-built survival technique, needed in the times when one never knew when a predator might appear, and we would need to fight or flee. So, what served us in historic times as a survival mechanism today works against us with the abundance of low-nutritional, high-glycaemic-index foods.

LOVE TRAINING YOUR BODY TO BURN FAT

When training at an optimum fat-burning zone, you will find that your enjoyment of exercise will be maintained. Burning body fat will keep you motivated, and recovery time will be short. The main benefit of exercising in your body-fat-burning zone is that you won't crave sugars at the end of the fat-burning workout. This exercise range will also help to flush toxins out of your system.

LOSE WEIGHT WHILE YOU SLEEP

Regular strength training helps build muscles and muscular endurance. Furthermore, it is now widely recognised that strength training is one of the most effective ways to reduce your body fat, control your weight and increase your muscle mass.

Logic commands that the more muscle mass you have, the more your body burns calories, even while at rest. Properly conditioned muscles are essential in carrying out everyday activities both at work and home, especially as we age and our muscles naturally tend to shrink due to lack of use and hormonal declines which we have already discussed.

A simple guideline to strength training is to do at least two sessions per week. In each session, include six to eight different exercises utilising the major muscle groups and work up to three sets of at least eight to 12 repetitions of each exercise.

As with any physical activity, warm up and cool down effectively. Most workout injuries can be avoided by a proper warm up and cool down.

You should start strength training on an appropriate level. If you begin the strength training at too high a level, you will risk injury and you also develop poor form and hinder your efforts and discourage yourself.

However, if you start out with too light a weight, and after many workouts you find you are not getting any gains at all. This will also disillusion you and you won't maintain your exercise program.

You also need to get proper instructions at first, to make sure that you have good technique to get the most effective workout out from your strength-training regime. This will also reduce your chance of injury and increase your enjoyment for lifting techniques.

Using proper lifting techniques will help your muscles through their full range of motion, by not locking any joints, lifting at a speed in which you can control the weight and easily stop if necessary, and maintain a good posture. You should never throw the weights around or lose control of any motion.

You should always try to exercise large muscle groups first. Exercise your chest, back and legs before exercising your biceps, triceps and small muscle groups. Your abdominals are considered by many to be a large muscle group, but they are actually a large muscle mass built up of small muscles. Train them last.

You should progress gradually, increasing your reps and your resistance. Reduce the rest intervals between sets, to increase the workload on your cardiovascular system at the same time.

You should also breathe correctly. Never hold your breath and exhale when you are doing the highest effort working a load. Muscles get built by shocking them out of complacency. You do this most effectively by varying and changing your exercise routine when training your different muscle groups.

All strength training should progress gradually, increasing your weight until your goals and plateaus are reached, then change your workout to include increased reps or a higher weight level at the ends of each set.

Alter the order of exercise that you perform and perform multiple sets, in order to maintain results or new goals.

Remember to always give your muscles and mind a rest.

You need to get the most out of your strength training and give your muscles at least 48 hours rest between strength training workouts, to recover and rebuild.

HOW TO MINIMISE RISK

Avoid risking your health. If an exercise has a degree of risk of injury that exceeds the potential benefit, it is better to be on the conservative side and avoid those exercises. Always seek advice from fitness professionals, for guidance regarding optimum exercise.

You should consult your medical practitioner before starting any exercise program, especially if you are over 40 and have potential risk factors, such as a history of heart disease, obesity, high blood pressure or osteoporosis or if you smoke.

TIPS FOR ENJOYING AN EXERCISE PROGRAM TO STAY YOUNG

- Commit to your body and mind for 21 days. After that, exercise will be an enjoyable lifestyle habit.
- Set realistic goals and objectives that are obtainable and measurable.
- Exercise within your target heart-rate zone to get optimum fat-burning results or cardiovascular conditioning.
- Add variety to your program to increase motivation.
- Train with your partner, friend or personal trainer.
- Maintain a regular warm up and cool down routine.
- Stretch after warm up and before beginning any workout program.

- Stretch completely after cool down.
- Drink plenty of water before, during and after workout. If you wait until you are thirsty, then you have waited too long.
- Avoid caffeine and alcoholic beverages especially before and after exercise.
- Increase the duration or intensity by no more than 5% from your previous workout as your body adapts.
- Increase your weights in a resistance-training program by no more than 5% from your previous workout.
- First increase duration, then increase intensity.
- Avoid overdoing it in hot or humid weather.
- Never work out if you don't feel well. Listen to your body, it usually knows best.
- Injuries are the most common reasons for quitting exercise, from exercising too aggressively, or trying to do too much too soon.
- Whatever activity you choose, proceed at your own pace. Don't overdo it.
- Keep it convenient. The best and optimum way of exercising is to keep it convenient and close to home. You may also choose to work out at your home, even watching your favourite TV show, or while you read.
- Keep the time of day consistent and make it a time that works for you.
- Plan ahead. By planning ahead and showing commitment, you are more likely to exercise on a regular basis.
- Seek out fitness professionals to guide you and empower you to the benefits of exercise and you will be more motivated to enjoy your workouts.

- Dress for success! Equip yourself with the proper workout gear and you will feel more comfortable and have a better training experience.

MODERATE EXERCISE EXTENDS YOUR LIFE

Harvard University studied 17,000 male alumni aged between thirty-five and seventy-four. Those groups who exercised most had the lowest death rates. (Physician in charge: Dr. Ralph Raffenberger.)

Exercise and nutrients strengthen old people

A 1994 study at the Human Nutrition Research Centre on Ageing in Boston showed men and women over the age of 63 gained significant muscle strength and increased mobility after only 10 weeks on a multi–nutrient and exercise program.

According to Waneen Spirduso, author of *Physical Dimensions of Ageing*, people who get involved in strength training have the opportunity to reverse many of the age-related deterioration processes that are observed in sedentary people.

Recent studies have also shown that exercise may fight mental ageing as well as physical ageing.

Section 11

THE ANT[...]
YOUR M[...]

HOW DO YO[...]

Without knowle[...]
ness and disea[...]
excused by [...]
Now [...]
history [...]
to [...]

WHAT YOU[...]

If at this point yo[...] good indication of you[...] longevity.

There has been much information provided in this book to educate and guide you, and you may now feel you are ready to begin.

To succeed on this revolutionary **Anti-ageing Diet** is really simple. It is a decision and a lifelong commitment to doing the right things for your self and your body each day.

THE 6 'MUSTS . . .' TO STAYING YOUNG

You must eat right (now you know how) following the guidelines provided.

You must manage and avoid stress as much as possible.

You must incorporate exercise into your daily routine.

You must supplement your food with vitamins and minerals.

You must ensure your hormone levels are balanced.

You must avoid consumption of pollutants and toxins.

OU WISH TO LIVE
OUR LIFE?

dge we are blind. The prevalence of sick-
se in our society today can be momentarily
claiming we just 'didn't know'.

here is no excuse! We can and must learn from
, and we now have the knowledge and technology
everse the damage we have done to our health and
uality of life.

We now have a choice. If we want to live in modern society, we can choose to do nothing and accept that age and diseases associated with age are inevitable. Or we can decide to make some changes and begin taking responsibility for our health and remove our reliance on traditional medicine to 'save us' when we get sick.

We have the know-how and ability to reverse the effects of ageing, and in so doing reduce the chance of us contracting such common diseases as cancer, heart disease, diabetes, stroke, Alzheimer's etc.

We can reclaim our body biochemistry, remove toxins, restore energy and vitality, look better, feel better and live long and healthy lives.

It is our choice today. We do not have to cash out and go to live with the Hunzas to enjoy long and healthy lives. We can learn to do this right here where we live.

Whether you live a long healthy life or one that is plagued with sickness and disease and which robs you of your zest for life and your family of many more years of your health and support, is up to you.

It is your choice today.

Please make the right choice!

'Some people try to achieve immortality through their offspring or their work. I prefer to achieve immortality by not dying.' — Woody Allen

THE BEGINNING

Thank you for buying **The Anti-Ageing Diet** and investing your time reading it to the end.

I have saved this special message for those of you that have travelled this far.

This is the end of this book, yet it is hopefully for you only the beginning – the beginning of a new age of enlightenment about you, your place in the world in relation to the things you do, think and the way you treat your body.

Some people may simply dismiss this 'stuff' and say this is all quackery and rubbish. These will not be uneducated people and probably be your own doctor. So be it – most people once thought the earth was flat and anyone who disagreed or proposed a new view of the world, was ostracised.

It takes courage to be different and to be a leader in any field of endeavour. Saving people from themselves is no different.

If you are convinced as I was that prevention is better than cure, and this is what this book is all about, then staying young and healthy will be easy for you. If you are not yet convinced, then all I ask is that you give this a try for a few months and see the difference for yourself. Don't listen to what others may tell you, it is your life and your future we are dealing with.

I have done this myself well before I wrote this book and have seen the spectacular results first hand, and now I continue to see the great results of the many hundreds of people I have been able to educate on Anti-ageing.

My only wish for you is to achieve both Health and Happiness.
Brian Sher

PS. If you feel you would like to contact me for any reason please feel free to email me at briansher@bigpond.com.au

Appendix

THE REDWOOD ANTI-AGEING CLINIC

The Redwood Anti-ageing Clinics are state-of-the-art facilities specifically designed for those who place a great value on their health and longevity. Its exclusive environment provides an opportunity to meet and consult with some of the world's most knowledgeable physicians and Anti-ageing specialists, trained to provide tailored, ethical, scientifically proven Anti-ageing, peak-performance and disease-prevention programs.

These centres are among the most advanced in the world and are on the cutting edge of science and biochemistry to provide safe, effective Anti-ageing solutions, using natural non-pharmaceutical products manufactured to the highest possible standards.

Please call 03 9826 6665

REVERSE OSMOSIS FILTERS

Please contact 03 9682 0299

REDUCE EMF EFFECTS ON THE BODY

Recognising the rapidly growing worldwide EMF pollution problem, Clarus Products has responded with a line of innovative products for advanced EMF protection. Clarus developed and validated its technology in collaboration with internationally recognised scientists from Stanford University and the University of California. Using different testing methods, Clarus products are shown to reduce stress levels by 30% to 70%, especially stress caused by EMF sources such as computers and mobile phones.

Independent testing has shown that the QLink products with Sympathetic Resonance Technology™ (SRT™) neutralize the potentially harmful effects of EMF. Working like a tuning fork for your energy, the QLink products align your body's energy to its optimum level.

QLink customers report there is a difference in their daily lives. They experience enhanced energies, mental clarity and alertness, more balanced emotions, improved overall performance, are calmer, more balanced, and sleep better.

For more information call 0412 400945

References

Bjorksten, J., 'Crosslinkage and the Ageing Process,' In Rockstein, M. (ed): *Theoretical Aspects of Ageing*, Academic Press, New York, 1974, p. 43.

Bjorksten, J., 'The Crosslinkage Theory of Ageing: Clinical Implications,' *Compr Ther* II:65, 1976.

Campanelli, Linda, C., Ph.D., 'Theories of Ageing,' *Theories and Psychosocial Aspects of Ageing*, (1) 3–13.

Finch, Caleb, E., *Longevity, Senescence, and the Genome*, University of Chicago Press, 1990.

Hayflick, L., 'Theories of Ageing,' in Cape, R., Coe, R., and Rodstein, M. (eds), *Fundamentals of Geriatric Medicine*, Raven Press, New York, 1983.

Hayflick, L., *How and Why We Age*, Ballantine Books, New York, 1994, pp. 222–262.

Kotulak, Ronald and Gorner, Peter, 'Calorie Restriction: Taking the lifespan to its limit,' *Ageing on Hold*, Tribune Publishing, 1992, pp. 52–57.

Martin, G.M., Sprague, C.A. and Epstein, C.J., 'Replicative Lifespan of Cultivated Human Cells,' *Lab Invest* 23:26, 1970.

Medvedev, Z., 'Possible Role of Lifespans of Differential Cells,' *Nature* 237:453, 1972.

Review of Biological Research in Ageing, Vol. 4, edited by Martin Rothstein, Wiley-Liss, 1990.

Rose, Michael R., *Evolutionary Biology of Ageing*, Oxford University Press, 1991.

Rosenfeld, Albert, *Prolongevity* II, Alfred A. Knopf, Inc., New York, 1985, 247–267.

Sharma, Ramesh, 'Theories of ageing,' *Physiological Basis of Ageing and Geriatrics*, CRC Press, Florida, 1994, 37–44.

Sonneborn, T., 'The origin, Evolution, Nature, and Causes of Ageing,' In Behnke, J., Fince, C., and Moment, G. (eds), *The Biology of Ageing*, Plenum press, New York, 1979, p. 341.

Warner, H.R., Butler, R.N., Sprott, R.C., and Scheider, E.L., *Modern Biological Theories of Ageing*, Raven Press, 1987.

Cowley, Geoffrey, 'Melatonin,' *Newsweek*, August 7, 1995, pp. 46–49.

Hughes, Patrick, 'The Hormone Whose Time Has Come,' *Hippocrates*, July–August 1994.

Kane, M.A., Johnson, A., and Robinson, W.A., 'Serum Melatonin Levels in Melanoma Patients After Repeated Oral Administration,' *Melanoma Research* 1994; 4: 59–65.

Kent, Saul, Life Extention Reports, 'How Melatonin Combats Ageing,' *Life Extension Magazine*, December 1995, pp. 10–27.

Lissoni, P., Meregalli, S., Barni, S., and Frigerio, F., 'A Randomized Study of Immunotherapy with Low-Dose Subcutaneous Interleukin-2 Plus Melatonin vs. Chemotherapy with Cisplatin and Etoposide as First-Line Therapy for advanced Non-Small Cell Lung Cancer,' *Tumori* 1994; 80: 464–67.

McAuliffe, Kathleen, 'Live 20 Years Longer, Look 20 Years Younger,' *Longevity*, October 1990.

Muller, J., Stone, P., and Braunwald, E. , 'Circadian Variation in the Frequency of Onset of Acute Myocardial Infarction.' *New England Journal of Medicine* 1985; 313–21: 1315–22.

Pierpaoli, Walter, and William Regelson, with Carol Colman, *The Melatonin Miracle*, Simon & Schuster, New York, 1995, pp. 29–30.

Reiter, R.J., et al., 'A Review of the Evidence Supporting Melatonin's Role as an Antioxidant,' *Journal of Pineal Research*, Volume 18, No. 1, pp. 1–11.

Reiter, Russell J., Ph.D., and Jo Robinson, *Melatonin*, Bantam Books, New York, 1995, pp. 40–41, 62–69; (9), 116–118.

Sahelian, Ray, M.D., 'Melatonin: The Natural Sleep Medicine,' *Total Health*, August 1995, Vol. 17, No. 4. p. 30 (3).

Zhdanova, I.V., Wurtman, R.J., and Schomer, D.L., 'Sleep-inducing Effects of Low Doses of Melatonin Ingested in the Evening,' *Clinical Pharmacology and Therâpeutics* 1995; 57: 552–558.

Ben-Nathan, D., et al., 'Protection by Dehydroepiandrosterone in Mice Infected with Viral Encephalitis,' *Archives of Virology*, 1991; 120: 263–271.

Brody, Jane, 'Restoring Ebbing Hormones May Slow Ageing,' *New York Times*, July 18, 1995, p. c3.

Coleman, D.L., et al., 'Effect of Genetic Background on the Therapeutic Effects of Dehydroepiandrosterone (DHEA) in Diabetes – Obesity Mutants in Aged Normal Mice,' *Diabetes*, 1984; 33: 26.

Coleman, D.L., et al., 'Therapeutic Effects of Dehydroepiandrosterone (DHEA) 'Therapeutic Effects of Dehydroepiandrosterone (DHEA) in Diabetic Mice,' *Diabetes*, 1982; 31: 830–833.

Cranton, Elmer, M.D., and James P. Frackelton, M.D., 'Take Control of your ageing,' *Alternative Medicine Digest*, Issue 8, pps. 23–28.

Cryer, Sibyl, 'New Music and Stress Reduction Technique Increase anti-Ageing Hormone-DHEA- Study says,' *Institute of heart-math*, July 19, 1995, pp. 1–2.

'DHEA Replacement Therapy,' *Life Extension Report*, Vol. 13, No. 9, September 1993, p. 67.

Fettner, Ann Giudici, 'DHEA Gets Respect,' *Harvard Health Letter*, Vol. 19, No. 9, July 1994.

Gaby, Alan R., M.D., 'DHEA: The Hormone That Does It All,' *Holistic*, Spring 1993, pps. 19–22.

Life Extension Events, 'DHEA Comes to the Mainstream,' *Life Extension Magazine*, September 1995, pps. 1–4.

Life Extension Events, 'DHEA Replacement therapy,' *Life Extension Magazine*, March 1, 1995, p. 4.

Life Extension Foundation, *The Physician's Guide to Life Extension Drugs*, 1994 Edition, pp. 46–55.

Nasman, R., et al., 'Serum dehydroepiandresterone sulfate in Alzheimer's Disease and in Multi-Infarct Dementia,' *Biological Psychiatry*, 1991, 30: 684–690.

Regelson, W., et al., 'Hormonal Intervention: "Buffer Hormones" or "State Dependency": The Role of Dehydroepiandrosterone (DHEA), Thyroid Hormone, Estrogen, and Hypophysectomy in Ageing,' *Annals of the New York Academy of Science*, 1988, 521: 260–273.

'A physician Gives His Opinion About the Entry of STH into the World of Bodybuilding,' *Flex*, June 1983, p. 76.

Barbul; 'Arginine and Immune Function,' *Nutrition* 6 (1): 53-60, (up-date on Immunonutrition Symposium Supplement; Jan/Feb 1990.

Ceda, G., Valenti, G., Butterini, U., Hoffmann, A.R., 'Diminished Pituitary Response to Growth Hormone-Releasing Factor in Ageing Male Rats,' *Endocrinology* 1986; 118: 2109–14.

Crist, D.M., Peake, G.T., Egan, P.A., Waters, D.L., 'Body Composition

Response to Exogenous GH during Training in Highly Conditioned Adults,' *Journal of Applied Physiology* 65: 579–584. 1988.

Donaldson, Thomas, Ph.D., *Life Extension Report*, April 1991, Vol. 11, No. 4, p. 32.

Dr. Julian Whitaker's Health & Healing, Vol. 5, No. 7, July 1995, pp. 4–5.

Howard, Ben, 'Growing Younger', *Longevity*, October 1992, p. 41.

Journal of the American Medical Association, March 18, 1988, Vol. 259, No. 11, p. 1703 (3).

Kelly, K., et al., 'Gh3 Pituitary Adenoma Cells Can Reverse Thymic Ageing in Rats,' Proceedings of the National Academy of Sciences, Vol. 83, p. 5663, 1986, cited in 'Longevity: A Fresh Shot of Life,' *Omni*, Vol. 1, No. 9, July 1987, p. 85.

Lawren, 'The hormone that Makes Your Body 20 Years Younger,' *Longevity*, October 1990, p. 34.

Lehrman, Sally, 'The Fountain of Youth?', *Harvard Health Letter*, June 1992, Vol. 17, No. 8, p. 1 (3).

Marcus R.G., Holloway, L., et al., 'Effects of Short-Term Administration of Recombinant Human Growth Hormone to Elderly People,' *J Clin Endocrinol Metab* 1990: 519–27.

Merimee, et al., 'Arginine Initiated Release of Growth Hormone: Factors Modifying the Response in Normal men,' *New England Journal of Medicine* 280(26): 1434–38 (1969).

Movie The Legend of
Bagger Vance.